Health and Social Care: Knowledge and Skills

Understanding and Helping People in Crisis

Health and Social Care Series
Series Editors: Sue Cuthbert, Jan Quallington and
Elaine Donnelly – all at the University of Worcester

This series of textbooks is aimed at students on Health and Social Care
Foundation Degree programmes in FE and HE institutions. However, the
books also provide short introductions to key topics for Common Foundation
Programme modules and will be suitable for first-year undergraduate courses
in a variety of Health and Social Care subject areas. Books in the series will
also be useful for those returning to practice and for overseas nursing students.
The series includes three types of textbook:

- Knowledge and Skills books;
- Theory and Practice books;
- Specialist books that cover specific professions, topics and issues.

All titles in the series will address the common elements articulated in
relevant sector skill frameworks such as, for example, Skills for Care, Skills for
Health, the NHS Knowledge and Skills Framework and the Code of Practice
for Social Care Workers.

Titles in the series include:
Understanding Research and Evidence-based Practice by Bruce Lindsay
ISBN 978 1 906052 01 0
Values for Care Practice by Sue Cuthbert and Jan Quallington
ISBN: 978 1 906052 05 8
Communication and Interpersonal Skills by Elaine Donnelly and
Lindsey Neville
ISBN: 978 1 906052 06 5
Interpersonal Skills for the People Professions Edited by Lindsey Neville
ISBN: 978 1 906052 18 8
Essential Study Skills for Health and Social Care Edited by Marjorie Lloyd
and Peggy Murphy
ISBN 978 1 906052 14 0
*Safe and Clean Care: Infection Prevention and Control for Health and
Social Care Students* by Tina Tilmouth with Simon Tilmouth
ISBN: 978 1 906052 08 9
Understanding and Helping People in Crisis by Elaine Donnelly,
Briony Williams and Tess Parkinson
ISBN 978 1 906052 21 8
*Work-based Learning and Practice Placement: A Textbook for Health and
Social Care* Edited by Graham Brotherton and Steven Parker
ISBN: 978 1 906052 12 6

Visit **www.reflectpress.co.uk** for more details on these titles.

Health and Social Care: Knowledge and Skills

Understanding and Helping People in Crisis

Elaine Donnelly, Briony Williams and
Tess Parkinson

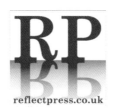

reflectpress.co.uk

First published in 2009

ISBN: 978 1 906052 21 8

British Library Cataloguing in Publication Data
A catalogue record for this book is available from the British Library

Production project management by Deer Park Productions
Typeset by Kestrel Data, Exeter, Devon
Cover design by Oxmed
Printed and bound in the UK by Bell & Bain Ltd, Glasgow

www.reflectpress.co.uk

Published by Reflect Press Ltd
11 Attwyll Avenue
Exeter
Devon, EX2 5HN
UK
01392 204400

Contents

Author Biographies

Elaine Donnelly

My main role is leading the Graduate Diploma Course in Mental Health Nursing at the University of Worcester but I teach across a range of health and social care programmes. My interests include mental health, psychology, communication skills and death, dying and bereavement. To maintain my clinical skills I offer a counselling and advice service to people living at a local YMCA hostel and as a personal tutor I support students who, like the rest of the population, experience all sorts of personal crisis.

Tess Parkinson

I currently work half-time in clinical practice, working as part of a small cognitive behavioural therapy (CBT) team within a Mental Health Trust, and half-time working in continuing professional development, mainly supporting growth of clinical supervision throughout the local Trusts, for a variety of health care professionals. I am also part of a team developing a Masters degree in psychological therapies. Previous teaching experiences include: NVQ Assessor and External Verifier, developing and delivering a staff nurse development programme, foundation counselling skills for statutory and voluntary services, contributing to training for voluntary workers in the private sector.

Briony Williams

My current role is Course Leader for Foundation Degrees and Pathway Leader for the Child and Adolescent Mental Health Foundation degree at the University of Worcester. I am also a member of the Applied Social Science teaching team. My main areas of teaching are mental health conditions, interventions in mental health, substance misuse and therapeutic group work. I have previously taught at Coventry University on the undergraduate BSc Hons in occupational therapy and the MSc in occupational therapy. My current clinical experience is working with young people with psychosis, in the past I have worked as an occupational therapist in community mental health services, substance misuse and acute mental health provision.

Chapter 1

Introduction: What is a crisis?

Key themes

This chapter introduces you to:

- the book in context;

- exploring a common understanding of crisis;

- crisis in the context of groups and nations;

- individual crisis;

- a new model for understanding crisis.

INTRODUCTION

It is likely that everyone, during the course of their lives, will experience times of crisis. A crisis, when it strikes, may affect lots of people such as in a public or national emergency, or it may be a private experience affecting only one individual or a family. During their lives some people experience more crises than others and, while many appear to manage very well, others really struggle to cope with the potential dangers that crisis presents, either to themselves or to their loved ones.

Crises can happen for all sorts of reasons and they come in many different guises. A crisis can happen to anyone regardless of who they are, where they are, or their health and personal circumstances. We, the authors, have spent our professional lives working with a wide variety of people, many of whom have experienced a broad range of crises. We would like to acknowledge those we have worked with over the years. We would also like to give special thanks to those who have more recently shared their personal stories of crises with us and many of their contributions are presented and analysed within this book. The stories and details presented here have been anonymised to protect the identity of those whom they concern, and it should be noted that all contributors gave their consent to use their experiences and some of them played an active part in the analysis of the outcomes.

Having analysed individual stories, our thoughts and ideas about how people survive crises have been validated and we offer here the culmination of those thoughts and present them in an easy-to-use framework for understanding what happens to people when they experience crisis. We identify key influencing factors that help determine the outcome of crisis and we offer a range of theoretical and practical strategies that have been identified as being useful in helping people cope. We also provide a range of valuable links to key resources that are readily available to anyone seeking help in the areas we discuss. The ultimate goal of the text is to equip you, as an individual, with an opportunity to review your skills and knowledge and enable you to cope more effectively with crisis situations – your own or those of other people.

THE BOOK IN CONTEXT

This chapter introduces the reader to the concept of crisis, touching upon global perspectives, local emergencies and personal experiences. This macro/micro perspective then sets the scene for exploring what crisis means to individuals within their personal and social experience. To illustrate common experiences a new model of crisis is presented, using the simple mnemonic FRAGILE TEARS. This model offers an easy-to-use diagrammatic illustration that represents the person and their social world and includes many of the key external influences on our lives.

Chapter 2 offers a review of personal stories that reflect a range of common personal crises encountered in ordinary everyday lives. The accounts are linked to the FRAGILE TEARS framework to enable a quick and easy understanding and each account includes activities to ensure a deeper level of learning. Chapter 2 explores the impact that outside influences have on an individual. At the end of each story we provide internet and, where available, telephone links to some of the key external agencies and resources that have been useful for people experiencing similar situations to those explored.

Chapter 3 introduces crisis theory and its origins. Grief reactions and determinants of grief are explored as an explanation of what happens to people in crisis, alongside the development of physiological theories of crisis. Psychoanalytical theories, coping and defence mechanisms and a transactional analysis perspective are explored within this chapter as well as an introduction to cognitive and behavioural understandings of what happens to people when a crisis occurs. Using examples from the accounts of personal crises in Chapter 2, this chapter enables the reader to map those theoretical perspectives against our model of crisis FRAGILE TEARS. This will help the reader to understand further how theory can be used in analysing crisis and how proven practical helping approaches are underpinned by theory.

Chapter 4 provides an overview of crisis interventions as well as the development of practical helping skills and the role of the crisis worker. The role of reflection, self awareness, communication skills and motivation are explored alongside the need to work within a legislative framework, the concept of ethical practice and the importance of working within role boundaries. By revisiting the personal narratives, the reader has an opportunity to implement their new knowledge and understanding and consider potential outcomes. The chapter concludes by offering a summary of healthy living strategies and provides more detail about contacts and resources that may be useful to individuals and to practitioners who are, as part of their role, helping people deal with crisis.

Chapter 5 goes on to review the potential outcomes of crisis. Positive and negative crisis resolutions and potential for recovery and change are explored. This final chapter includes the more serious outcomes of crisis including post-traumatic stress disorder, mental illness and the risk of suicide, alongside the potential for recovery and change. The book concludes with the importance of debriefing, working together and looking after the self.

Studying with this book

As you read through each chapter you will be invited to supplement your reading with a variety of activities that will involve you in reflecting on your experiences or on what you already know. Reflection can be a powerful tool in enabling you to make sense of a given situation or theoretical perspective. Jasper (2003) explores the concept of reflective practice in nursing, health and social care and offers a range of reflective models that may be useful to you. For further detail and models of reflection, you can visit **www.reflectivepractice.com**. This website offers some valuable tools for reflection alongside some worked examples that will help you to make sense of your thoughts and actions. The activities may ask you to put yourself in the place of others and to practise achieving an empathic understanding (seeing the world as others see and experience it to be). This is done to emphasise particular points and appreciate the wider perspective. Where online or telephone facilities are available we will provide you with a website address and/or telephone number that was current at the time of writing and you are encouraged to follow these links.

This book is just like any other in that it is full of detail and ideas for further study but it is the reader that can make it come alive and work. You are encouraged to jot down notes as you read and you may wish to annotate the text to indicate how helpful the resources are and what you can do to further supplement your study. Whatever helps you to learn is encouraged and we trust that you will find this book informative and, more importantly, helpful in how you support others through their crisis and also in dealing with personal crisis.

EXPLORING A COMMON UNDERSTANDING OF CRISIS

Take some time to identify your own thoughts about what constitutes a crisis.

Activity

- How would you define a personal crisis?
- What sorts of common personal crises do people have?
- It may be useful to list your key points and share them with another person to see if your responses are similar.

In our developed nation, Western and European lives we probably share an understanding of what constitutes a 'common crisis'. Marriage or relationships ending, unemployment, serious illness, facing disability and even sudden death are all common experiences that we are likely to describe as 'a crisis'. The *Collins Dictionary* (2000) defines crisis as '1. a crucial stage or turning point . . . 2. an unstable period . . . 3. a sudden change, for better or worse . . . from the Latin to decide'. This definition suggests that when in a crisis, change is enforced upon us or that we have to make a decision to change so as to avoid a worsening situation. Perhaps this definition goes some way to summarise and embrace some of your key points. Parry (1990) outlines her definition of crisis in a similar manner but she adds that there are 'other layers of meanings', suggesting that crisis is a personal experience that is subject to what is meaningful to us.

We use the word 'crisis' in everyday conversation to explain our own personal circumstances and to describe stressful situations, but what constitutes a crisis for one person may not affect another. Parad (1965) supports this notion and suggests that 'the crisis is not the situation itself but the person's perception of it'. How we perceive crisis goes some way to explain why there are such differences in how people cope, or not, with the same or similar crisis but, as we all experience personal crisis, there are some events that impact on groups of people at the same time.

Crisis in the context of groups and nations

Families may share a crisis when something happens to them such as serious illness; communities may experience a crisis as a result of a local disaster such as heavy rain and localised flooding; and nations may experience a crisis, for example, as seen in the Sudan and the repeated failure of crops and adverse weather. News headlines use the term 'crisis' as one that is interchangeable with other terms such as disaster, emergency and tragedy. We 'Googled' the word 'crisis' in an open, general web-based search and we received 170,000,000 hits. That figure represents an awful lot of individual, group and corporate views on crisis.

Activity

Try doing your own internet search and review the range of commentary, products and people who offer their thoughts and opinions on crisis. You can narrow down your search by adding additional target words such as 'personal' or 'global' and you can narrow that down further by including relevant words such as 'divorce' or 'depression'.

You will see that the word 'crisis' is used on many levels and in our study we became aware of the macro and micro perspectives, that is the big and the smaller picture of crisis. Although this book is fundamentally about individuals and, in the main, focuses on micro (personal) perspectives, it would be amiss not to give mention to the terrible crises we see on a macro/global level that others refer to, as each can be seen to influence our lives in some way.

For example, the financial and political crisis our world faces in 2009 will change our lives regardless of our position or status. Some will benefit and others will not. Every rise or fall in interest rates, threats to our pension or mortgage rates becomes a banner headline. As the media coverage of the current financial crisis is reinforced, it becomes more personal to us as we see our local businesses and shops closing down. The financial recession and how we live in local communities make us more than likely to know someone who is under threat or has been made redundant. Unsurprisingly, according to Ogden (2007), actual or threatened loss of income has a negative effect on our stress levels and consequently money worries may push some individuals beyond their coping ability. Economic crisis has an impact on our lives and on our health. Depression, increased irritability, hostility, aggression, anxiety and somatic complaints are all possible reactions to reduction in working hours or redundancy. Sadly, children and young people, who are about to embark on adult life and meet with the responsibilities that adulthood brings, are also embroiled in the social after-effects of financial distress. The Enterprising Rural Families Newsletter (2005) mentions possible effects that economic crisis has on our young people, such as:

- fear of the future;
- loss of peer status;
- deterioration in academic performance;
- feeling isolated from family and friends;
- risk of acting-out behaviour.

Activity

Take a moment to reflect on how you and your family's life would be affected by the loss of your job (or the job of another member of your family).
- Are there things you would have to give up or reduce?
- How do you think you would manage?
- How would others in your social circle react?
- How would you feel about yourself?

Work is not only a place for earning money; it also feeds our self-esteem and affects our beliefs about who we are. The questions we may have to consider here are linked to who we are, our purpose in life and how we get refreshment in our lives. Work, or having a meaningful role to play in life, gives us the energy to continue and significantly enhances the opportunity for us to find enjoyment and fulfilment from our lives.

According to some researchers, we are facing an even bigger crisis that is far more important than money or politics – and that is climate change and global warming. Regardless of whether the theory of global warming is accurate, we do know that extremes of weather affect individuals, communities, towns and cities across the world and regularly result in crisis for many people. That people and communities survive ecological disasters such as cyclones, hurricanes, tsunamis, flooding, fire and drought, let alone the ravages of war, poverty and extreme deprivation, serves as a reminder of the resilience of human beings and our ability to rebuild our lives. As an example of the extreme conditions that people survive you may wish to follow the web link in the next exercise. The link gives you an opportunity to see the impact of Cyclone Nargis 2008, one of the biggest cyclones ever recorded, and you can view the conditions that people have to live in, you can hear the survivors' stories and see how they are continuing to rebuild their lives.

Activity

Visit the web link: **http://geology.com/events/cyclone-nargis** and try to imagine yourself in the same situation as the people you can see on your computer screen.
- What would your thoughts and feelings be, experiencing this disaster?
- Alternatively, how would you feel if some of those people were related to you?

It may be that you found the exercise difficult. The situation in Burma is so alien to our own experiences here in the Western world. The cyclone resulted in the death of many people, leaving survivors in a situation where they had no power, no food, no clean water, no shelter and their safety was severely compromised. Cyclone Nargis, like many other natural disasters, left the local population with grief, trauma, helplessness and life-threatening disease. However, experience has shown that, despite the most extreme hardship, human life goes on.

Emergency planning

Before we leave this macro perspective it is useful to know that government and charitable organisations all have emergency plans to respond to such crises. Many of these agencies respond in a practical way and organise and co-ordinate the delivery of first emergency aid that includes the supply of fresh water, nutrition, shelter and medical supplies, taking care of basic human needs. The Inter-Agency Standing Committee of the World Health Organisation has also produced 25 Action Sheets that issue guidelines detailing mental health and psychosocial support in emergency settings.

Activity

Visit the following web address and read about what support is to be made available in a state of emergency. **www.humanitarianinfo. org/iasc/content/products/default.asp** or, alternatively, you can email them with any specific questions you may have at **IASCmhpss@who.int**

In the UK local government is required by law under the Civil Contingencies Act 2004 to have a major emergency plan in place ready to respond to the nature of the emergency. More details available at **www. direct.gov.uk/en/governmentcitizensandrights/index.htm**

If you are unfortunate enough to have been affected by a local emergency you will have seen and perhaps experienced the response of the emergency services and other agencies such as hospitals, community services, parish councils, voluntary services, local transport providers, local energy providers and the military, all co-ordinated by a local emergency centre that is ready to respond to a phone call. Take a look at your local emergency plan that is available either at your local library or via the web link given above by adding your locality to the search option, and see how the process works.

Golan (1978) commented that 'crisis situations occur episodically during the normal life span of individuals, families, groups and nations' and he identified a crisis as being a situation in which decisions have to be made to prevent a worsening situation. Golan's work acknowledges that crisis happens to us all and he suggests that all crises need to be thought through carefully and responded to on a 'needs must' basis. This principle can be applied to individuals, families, groups and nations but, when attempting to respond to crisis situations, it is important to remember there is no 'magic wand' to cure all and that some situations may get worse. Emergency plans and world aid seek to address the basic needs of people in order to make sure they survive.

In your work situation if you are helping people cope with personal crisis you may be involved in helping on many levels from meeting basic needs to enabling people to resolve their difficulties. It has been interesting to hear that many people, when facing personal adversity, compared their lives with the lives of others whom they considered to be much less fortunate than themselves. In times of trouble people reported that they found some comfort in 'counting their blessings' and that this helped them put their lives into perspective.

Experiencing individual crisis

Having briefly discussed community, national and world crises, we return now to focus on the individual. Here are some of the unique definitions of crisis offered to us by ordinary people when we asked them the question 'what does personal crisis mean to you?'

> A crisis is when something totally unexpected happens to you and you have to do something really quick to stop it from getting worse . . .

> Not being in the right place at the right time and losing something that is really important because of it . . .

> Being mugged in broad daylight and nobody caring enough to stop and help . . .

> When your world falls apart and all you can do is stand and watch . . .

> Finding out your husband is having an affair . . .

> Being out of control and having to rely on others to save your son's life . . .

> Finding yourself no longer able to take care of yourself and having to give up your home to go into a nursing home . . .

> Having a seizure in the middle of the night at the age of 36. I lost my licence, my job and it nearly cost me my marriage . . .

> Getting kicked out for something you haven't done . . .

> Having your home destroyed by stinking flood water . . .

When someone you really love dies . . .

When the baby that you waited for, for so long, was born with disabilities . . .

Cancer . . .

This list of responses may appear quite shocking in its entirety but all of these things have happened to ordinary people leading ordinary lives. Through our work with people who have experienced personal crisis and through our research we have identified the following themes.

- Crisis is often unexpected.
- Crisis can be the result of a series of events and therefore be considered inevitable.
- Crisis can be an individual/family/communal/cultural/national experience but it impacts on people in different ways.
- Crisis triggers deep feelings and emotions in people and often leads to a disruption and disorganisation of self.
- People in crisis experience a sense of being helpless and out of control.
- Crisis demands decisions and forces change.
- The aftermath of crisis can go on for a considerable period of time.
- Crisis can result in a strengthening of coping abilities and makes some people stronger.
- Sometimes people don't ever fully recover from the crisis experienced.

Activity

Considering the social world and environment in which you live and the people that you know, what would you identify as the common thought patterns and emotions of someone in crisis?

While people's reactions to crisis vary, it is likely that you were able to identify common recognisable thought patterns and emotions of people in crisis. For example, people experiencing crisis often report going over and over the event in their minds, trying to make sense of what is happening to them. They may question their own spiritual and religious beliefs and the existence of their god or deity, they may question why this is happening to them, questioning the fairness of it all in relation to the sort of person they believe themselves to be. Bad things happen to good people all the time. Some people report having nightmares; not being able to escape their thoughts through sleep. Many have hostile thoughts about the situation and may feel angry towards other people who were involved in the crisis such as, for example, doctors in the case of an illness. Many people report feeling overwhelmed by their emotions and having a sense of being completely alone when facing crisis, and all of the people we spoke to expressed a sense of denial, the hope that the crisis would just go away and that life would somehow revert to normal.

Activity

Consider the following questions:
- Do people revert back to normal after a crisis?
- For how long is a situation a crisis?
- How can we best help those in crisis?

Reverting back to normal is what we all seek at times of crisis but life will never be the same again as the crisis influences and shapes the person who experiences it. There may be resolution and a new beginning following a crisis or there may be a continued grief that lives with us for evermore. The aftermath of crisis may be much more serious and impact on the mental health of the individual, possibly resulting in post-traumatic stress disorder or even resulting in self-harm and suicide (these outcomes to crisis are dealt with in more detail in Chapter 5).

Even if we consider the crisis to have stages, such as the acute crisis and post-acute crisis stages, the question 'when does a crisis end?' is difficult to ascertain. Parad (1965) suggests a two- to six-week period before we experience a sense of getting back to normal after an acute crisis but it surely must be determined by the nature of the crisis and how it affects us, not least how we define and perceive the crisis and its outcomes. Perhaps we can only fully understand the impact of crisis on others when it has a significant impact on us, but what we can do to help those in crisis is to develop our understanding and empathy skills.

INTRODUCING THE 'FRAGILE TEARS' MODEL OF CRISIS

To illustrate what happens to people before, during and after crisis we have designed the following model to help aid your understanding. Based on a stage approach, there are three illustrations: Figure 1 representing a pre-crisis stage, Figure 2 representing the crisis stage and Figure 3 representing the post-crisis stage.

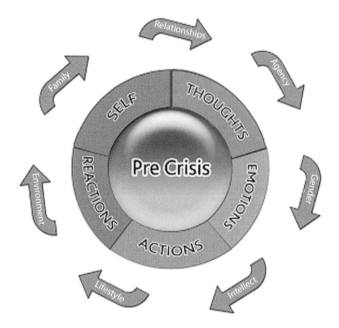

Figure 1 Pre-crisis stage

The pre-crisis stage

The pre-crisis stage of everyday living is represented by the illustration provided as Figure 1. The illustration is intended to represent the whole person who is not yet in crisis. The inner circle in the model represents our Thoughts, Emotions, Actions and Reactions which are unique to our Self (TEARS). In an ordinary healthy state our thoughts and emotions are in harmony and they are congruent with who we are. For example, we can actively direct our thoughts to the thing we have in focus at the time, be it writing a letter, collecting a parcel from the sorting office, doing the Sunday crossword or thinking about what to wear tomorrow. Our thoughts and perceptions of the world are clearly involved in how we assess a situation and, subject to our thoughts, our actions can then be seen as being rational and in keeping with our selves. For example, taking action to collect the parcel from the sorting office requires some thought about how to get there, checking when the office is open and where you can park the car, etc.

Just as we can undertake planned action, we can also show reactions to situations without thinking. We laugh out loud, sometimes to others' detriment and sometimes just because we can and, when caught unaware, we show our pleasure or our disdain to people around us. Reactions are often a display of our emotional state at the time. With regard to our emotions we can be sad, angry or frightened and react accordingly, as well as take a thoughtful action without calling it a crisis. Overall, when we are healthy and not in crisis, our thoughts, emotions, actions and reactions are harmonious and congruent within the world in which we live.

Around the inner circle of the illustrated model are arrows flowing in what can be seen as a comfortable clockwork direction, representing those outside factors that influence who we are, how we think, how we feel and how we behave. We offer the following detail as an overview of each arrow.

Family and friends

This relates to the people we are linked with through family structures, kinship and close relationships. This may include the nuclear family, i.e. parents and their children; the extended family, i.e. those relatives that sit outside the nuclear family unit but are in some way genetically connected such as grandparents, uncles, aunts and cousins; and reconstituted families i.e. where another family unit exists through ties as, for example, in divorce and re-marriage. As such, the family may not conform to our stereotype. Sociologists have long debated the role of the family in industrialised society and, in particular, the place of women and children within a family unit (Allan, 1985; Jamieson, 1998) as well as the role of intimacy and emotional attachment. The role that we have within our families will influence how we respond and behave within our world and, in part, determines our sociological role elsewhere. Alongside these relationships are the ties we have with our friends, those people to whom we may have a close intellectual or emotional bond.

Relationships

This component refers to the relationships we have with those who affect our lives but who are not related to us or held as close friends. For example, our manager, teacher or the people we work with can all influence who we are and how we think and behave. We meet people on a daily basis and, although the relationship may appear to be superficial such as, for example, the man in the canteen or the woman on reception, the relationship may take on a significant role when we find ourselves in a crisis. As users of various services we develop relationships with volunteers, people in similar circumstances and professionals and each one of them may go on to play an important part in helping us deal with crisis. Relationships are an important part of our everyday structure as we all seek contact with others. Transactional analysis, as outlined by Donnelly and Neville (2008), offers a simple approach to understanding how we all need the recognition of others and how we all need contact with others to be the person we are. There are clearly many different types of relationships, and how we manage or use these relationships, whether they are mutually respectful or not, all affect our responses to the world.

Agencies

Just as we are individuals so we are also part of the structure of the society in which we live and the structure of society in turn influences what we do. As individuals we have the ability to change but change on a societal level is limited to what people will allow and what is available. This is a complex construct that you may wish to follow further. For our purposes we identify agencies to be those organisations and structures that we may belong to, or that may impact on our lives. For example, the NHS, local facilities, local and national government, education and voluntary agencies. You might work for one of these agencies and use them at the same time. For example, you may be a receptionist at a local health centre and you may also use the services offered there. Within the agencies we use we may also develop relationships with specific individuals. However, there are many agencies that most people do not come into direct contact with at any stage in their lives. If we don't have a house fire we won't need the fire service; if we don't have legal problems we won't need lawyers or citizens advice bureaux; but indirect contact is inevitable. Consider the outcome if society did not have emergency services and what life would be like without the law.

Gender

Our sex is biologically determined for us, i.e. male and female, but our gender is said to be socially created and includes both masculine and feminine traits. Who we are sexually impacts upon every aspect of our everyday experience. Our gender identity, sexual orientation and sex role stereotypes that identify some aspects of behaviour to be either feminine or masculine exist in almost every culture (Williams and Best, 1990). Women are portrayed as soft-hearted and weak while men are associated with strength and aggression. In many cultures women are seen as possessions and must do as their elders or parents demand. Males, who are seen as the stronger, dominant sex, make major decisions that impact on women's lives. For example, forced marriages and to some extent arranged marriages are decided upon by family traditions that are upheld by the head of the household, i.e. the man. Our sexual orientation affects the life we live and the normalisation of each aspect is reflected in the services and the agencies available to us at times of crisis. Women's role in society is often under scrutiny and feminist theory suggests that women are socially disadvantaged in what is seen as a male-dominated world.

Intellect and information

The information that is available to us and the level of intellect required to understand that information plays a big part in our lives. If asked a question by a six-year-old it is hoped that our response would be in keeping with their level of understanding and, similarly, if a mature adult asks a question we respond accordingly. Information needs to be clear, understandable and meaningful to the recipient. Useful information is sometimes hard to find and information that is available is not always helpful. The ten-year census for Great Britain undertaken in 2001 was translated into 24 languages to ensure that the majority of the population were served with a questionnaire that was understandable. Language can be a major source of additional stress for people experiencing crisis and lack of understanding can and does worsen situations. The development of the internet has resulted in a great deal of information being readily available at the click of a mouse but that information is not necessarily accurate. Finding *bona fide* websites can be difficult but once found they can be invaluable to the individual seeking help and support. Information is power and helpers may need to consider how best to access and deliver information, subject to the ability of the person to understand the format in which the information comes.

Lifestyle

The authors have taken lifestyle to embrace the concepts of culture, occupation and economics. Culture can include whatever holds us together as groups, communities and societies and there are many definitions. We therefore took the following definition as the one that best represented our views on culture: 'Culture in its broadest sense is cultivated behaviour that is the totality of a person's learned, accumulated experience which is socially transmitted' (**www.tamu.edu/classes/cosc/ choudhury/culture.html**).

We learn how to behave in accord with our culture and we are expected to abide by our cultural heritage. Values and beliefs that are passed down to us through our families include religious beliefs, language, customs, rites and rituals. The way we dress, our manners and etiquette are all guided by our cultural experience. We live in what is described as a multicultural society where different cultures live alongside each other. At their best, different cultures coexist but there are times when cultural differences can result in tension and crisis situations can ensue.

How we fill our time every day, whether we are working or not, whether we are engaged in a meaningful activity in our lives or not, plays a part in shaping who we are and how we function. Our occupation may bring a source of prestige that reflects our personal values and those of society. For example, to work for the public sector can be viewed as a good thing and within that your position in the public sector will hold some prestige. The consultant paediatrician may have high prestige whereas the ward cleaner may have a low prestige and the unemployed have no prestige at all but this is clearly subject to your perspective. The role of working mums is often debated and political policy has encouraged mothers to take an active part in the workforce, but the effects on children are under scrutiny, thus creating a dilemma for the individual and society at large. Within our occupation there will be set rules as well as hidden ones and some occupations bring with them advantages such as flexitime and working at home, which enable people to manage some difficulties as they arise. For others their occupation dictates that they must be present at the job and there is no flexibility at all.

Alongside occupation we need to consider economics. Economics and the economic institutions intrinsically linked to our personal finances all play a key part in our lives. Whether or not we can pay for bare essentials or luxuries plays a big part in our lives, ranging from what we eat to how we entertain ourselves. Linked to occupation, economics influence personal choice and freedom and the financial position of our society influences what can be made available to us. Living in a wealthy Western country is very different to living in the developing world.

Environment

Finally the arrow that represents our environment includes our home and the place where we live. Home can be a mansion or a shelter and anything in between. Our home can be anywhere in the world and subject to the variances of nature and geography as well as those things relating to possession and occupation. The household is a diverse concept. Some people live alone, others live with families, while others live with friends and some find themselves sharing facilities with strangers. Home can be a secure place or hostile one. It is clear that a person's home will influence and be influenced by many things and plays a key role in our lives.

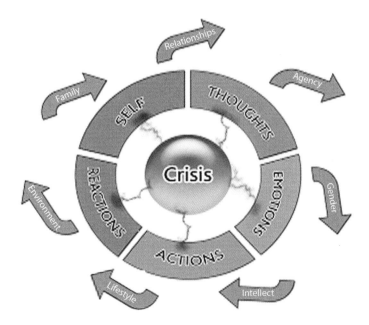

Figure 2 The FRAGILE TEARS model of crisis

The crisis stage

As crisis hits us there is seen to be a disorganisation and disruption in who we are and how we behave. The crisis stage, illustrated in Figure 2, depicts thoughts, emotions, actions, reactions and the sense of self being hit by crisis. The force of crisis can be so strong as to make us feel unattached from our normal self. This sense of disconnectedness is common in people who experience crisis. People who have had a crisis use descriptive terms such as: 'being shattered'; 'being blown apart'; 'blown away'; 'hit with a sledgehammer'; 'being broken', and 'totally losing control' to describe their experience. When we are in crisis we find ourselves thinking and feeling and reacting in ways that are unfamiliar to our normal selves. We have represented this experience in Figure 2 as bolts of lightning that appear to strike at the very core of the person.

When the crisis stage occurs people describe extreme thoughts and emotions such as intense fear, despair and often anger aimed either at the self, for having missed something and not having taken action to avert the situation, or aimed at other people who may be perceived to be responsible for the situation. People often experience overwhelming feelings of anxiety or a numbness that prevents them from functioning in their normal way.

Actions and reactions during crisis can be out of keeping with the normal presentation of self. There may be arguments, raised voices and expressions of despair underpinned often by misunderstandings and made in the heat of the moment. There may possibly be some personal history attached to some of the reactions displayed and feelings and thoughts that have been previously kept to oneself spill out all of a sudden in an uncontrolled and potentially damaging way. People repeat reactions under crisis and patterns of behaviour can become established as a response to stress that are not conducive to positive coping strategies. Shouting at loved ones, pushing people away, rejecting help and screaming at others are all common reactions to crisis.

Alongside this we may see people move into automatic behaviours such as making tea and it is not unusual to see people undertake activities that appear a little odd, such as choosing to go shopping for what appear to be trivial items but often reflect a meaningful action that brings comfort to a dire situation.

During crisis periods thoughts are often in turmoil and sometimes may not make any sense. Thoughts may be obsessive in nature as people ruminate over particular aspects of the crisis, planning and trying to problem-solve but not able to take action. Reasoned actions that would normally have been conducted with ease, such as making contact with an external agency or seeking help, may become difficult as thoughts are affected by the crisis situation. This disjointedness can be experienced as a sense of the world 'being against me' and everyday activities being difficult to manage. This situation is represented in Figure 2 by the disruption of those external influences in the crisis stage.

Reflection

Refer back to your visit to the website about the people who experienced the devastating hurricane in Burma.

- How might the outer circle of the model be affected as a result of this emergency situation?
- Can you identify similarities with the personal crises of people you have reflected upon?
- As a helper, how might you set about assisting a person in crisis in both situations?

Crisis brings with it a demand to change. That change can be recognisable by the situation being amended or reversed as, for example, if a couple that split up got back together again or the child that was ill became well again, or by a change in the person's perspective. As people change their perspective they re-evaluate the situation and the key role in helping people in crisis is to help them meet their needs and assist them in dealing with the consequences of crisis.

Many people expressed to us that, after a time, they realised they had to get used to the situation, they had to adjust and get used to their new experience, learning to live with it and take charge again rather than react against it. Personal crisis is said to be time-limited and that we should expect to see an individual changing their perspective and functioning again within a six-week period (Parry, 1990) but there is no doubt that after a crisis has abated there are often emotional scars that may take longer to heal.

The post-crisis stage

This scarring is illustrated in Figure 3 offered as the post-crisis stage. This illustration depicts a very similar picture to the pre-crisis model. However, the lines created when thoughts, feelings, actions and reactions split apart during the crisis are still evident like scar tissue or a piece of mended pottery. While those disjointed sections are mended and appear to be back together, the scars remain.

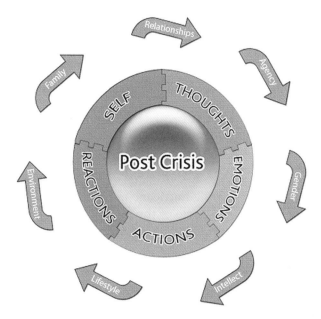

Figure 3 Post-crisis stage

As with fractures and mended pots these joins are different and sometimes tougher than they were in the pre-crisis stage but often they are vulnerable fractures that run the risk of being damaged again. There is no doubt in our view that crisis changes people. When reflecting on a crisis many people recognise that if it had never happened many other positive events would not have taken place and that they are in some way changed for ever: perhaps stronger, maybe more vulnerable but change has been seen to have taken place. The following chapters explore crisis on a personal level and examine the theories and models that attempt to explain crisis. Interventions and crisis-management strategies will be discussed alongside real people's stories about what was helpful in their time of crisis. We offer suggestions on how to judge when personal crisis becomes overwhelming and threatens people's mental health and personal safety, and provide information about a range of resources that are available to help.

REFERENCES

Allan, G. (1985) *Family Life*. Oxford: Blackwell

Collins Dictionary (2000)

Donnelly, E. and Neville, L. (2008) *Communication and Interpersonal Skills*. Exeter: Reflect Press

Enterprising Rural Families Newsletter (2005) **www.ageconuwyo.edu/ families/.../2005_02_NEWSLETTER**

Golan, N. (1978) *Treatment in Crisis Situation*. New York: Basic Books

Jamieson, L. (1998) *Intimacy*. Cambridge: Polity Press

Jasper, M. (2003) *Foundations in Nursing and Health Care: Beginning Reflective Practice*. Cheltenham: Nelson Thornes

Ogden, J. (2007) *Health Psychology* (4th edn). Maidenhead: Open University Press

Parad, A. (1965) 'A framework for studying families in crisis'. *Social Work Today*, 5 (3): 3–15

Parry, G. (1990) *Coping with Crisis*. The British Psychological Society in association with Routledge Press

Williams, J.E. and Best, D.L. (1990) *Measuring Sex Stereotypes: A Multi National Study*. Newbury Park: Sage Press

Useful websites

www.reflectivepractice.com

www.humanitarianinfo.org/iasc/content/products/default.asp

www.tamu.edu/classes/cosc/choudhury/culture.html

http://geology.com/events/cyclone-nargis/

www.direct.gov.uk/en/governmentcitizensandrights/index.htm

Chapter 2

Personal experiences of crises

Key themes

This chapter introduces you to personal experiences of crises including:

- childhood illness and negative outcomes;

- ending relationships;

- illness in adulthood;

- accidents and disability;

- financial debt and imprisonment;

- death and dying.

INTRODUCTION

This chapter details the experiences of people who agreed to take part in our exploration of personal crises. As each account is presented you will be invited to analyse specific detail that will require you to refer back to the FRAGILE TEARS model of crisis as presented in Chapter 1. It is important to remember that personal crisis is defined by the person experiencing it and the stories here vary from what you might judge to be a minor normal event in everyday life through to life-threatening illness and death.

Our sincere thanks go to those people who shared their stories with us and we wish to make clear that the stories used represent personal perspectives and may be viewed differently by others involved. Names have been changed along with other details to ensure anonymity but each person has consented to us using their story to help others understand what happens to our thoughts, feelings, actions, reactions and physical self when confronted with a crisis. These stories come from ordinary people and we present them in the hope that you will be able to relate to them either on a personal level or as someone working to help people in crisis. In later chapters theories, helping strategies and interventions will be introduced, enabling you to develop your understanding and skills in dealing with crisis.

The first two stories are about coping with childhood illness and facing the reality of the outcomes of serious illness.

ELLIE'S STORY

Ellie is a successful 35-year-old single mother who works full time. Ellie's daughter, Mae, was five months old, and being cared for by a childminder when she became unwell. Ellie describes how, over a period of three weeks, her daughter's condition did not appear to improve despite several visits made to the GP and the local Accident and Emergency department (A&E). Mae's symptoms were said to be possibly due to a lactose intolerance accompanied by a viral infection but, as Mae did not appear to get any better, the GP referred her to a specialist paediatric A&E for assessment. Mae was admitted to hospital, prescribed a course of antibiotics and eventually discharged home.

Several weeks later family members noticed that Mae still did not appear to be well, that she was unable to hold her head up and that she was exhibiting some odd movements. Ellie sought the advice of a health visitor who, on assessing Mae, insisted that she go back to the GP. As a result Mae was then referred to a neurologist and diagnosed with hydrocephalus.

It was said that this condition was likely to have been caused by a meningococcal infection that had not been treated adequately. Mae had to undergo a surgical procedure to have a shunt, which is a special drainage tube, inserted into her brain to drain away the excess fluid and relieve the inter-cranial pressure. Following surgery Mae appeared to recover well but on the next family visit Ellie's concerns about Mae's health were raised again.

While enjoying an extended family get-together, other babies became very upset at the sudden loud barking of a dog but Mae did not appear to respond to this very loud noise. There followed another referral to specialists and after testing it became apparent that Mae had a profound hearing impairment.

Activity

Ellie's story spans several months during which there appear to be a series of events that could be described as crises. Using your judgement identify, list and provide a short rationale of what you believe to be the crisis periods.

Ellie's story contains several episodes that had the potential for causing a personal crisis. Compare the following points with your responses.

The onset of Mae's illness

Ellie was in the process of adjusting to motherhood, trying to manage her return to work and leaving her daughter with a childminder. This period of adjustment can be very difficult for all parents, and particularly for single parents, and child illness can upset all childcare and work arrangements.

The GP's referral of Mae to a specialist paediatrician

This signals that the GP was still concerned about Mae's health.

The initial hospitalisation of Mae and the prescribed antibiotic treatment

When such a small child is admitted to hospital there is likely to be a great deal of anxiety. Many parents express distress at seeing their children exposed to testing and examination by the medical profession.

The family's comments about Mae's odd behaviour

Ellie had thought that Mae had recovered from her illness and to hear her family's comments that she appeared odd and was not achieving the expected developmental milestones was cause for great concern.

The diagnosis of hydrocephalus and the need for surgery

Hydrocephalus is a very serious condition in which there is an excessive amount of fluid in the cavities of the brain. The outcome of this condition could be brain damage and, untreated, hydrocephalus can be life-threatening. For an eight-month-old baby to undergo brain surgery is beyond most people's comprehension. Mae was in hospital for several days and Ellie never left her side. It must have been very difficult for her to watch her beautiful daughter develop this condition and then watch her undergo surgical treatment.

The family's recognition that despite all treatment Mae was still 'not right' and that she did not respond to loud noise

Ellie was again placed in a situation where other people's concerns alerted her to Mae still not being as she should be. Mothers are expected to make judgements about what is normal and what to expect of their children. For many mothers this knowledge comes with experience and via family and friends alongside other supportive networks and agencies. For new mothers finding out about parenting and being responsible for another human being is an enormous responsibility that has the potential to create a great deal of distress.

The diagnosis of profound deafness

There can be no doubt that this diagnosis will have had a huge impact on Mae's life and that of her mother.

All of these events have the potential for creating a personal crisis for Ellie but she presents as a strong woman who is able to cope with what appears to be very difficult circumstances. Using the FRAGILE TEARS model of crisis we are able to identify where Ellie's strength to cope under such difficult circumstances lies.

Ellie's perspective

Ellie is able to articulate what she believes to be the influencing factors involved in how she responded to the events as they occurred. When Mae was first ill Ellie describes her thoughts and feelings as being quite rational and under control. Ellie believes she took appropriate action, avoiding reactions that had not been thought through. She kept calm and trusted Mae's doctors and the treatment that they prescribed. Ellie is an intelligent woman, well educated and economically independent. Her employer was happy for her to manage her workload around Mae's needs, her family were supportive and knowledgeable and Ellie used a childminder whom she trusted explicitly. Even when Ellie found out that her daughter had a much more serious illness than originally thought and that she needed to have brain surgery, she says she was still able to cope with the situation and she describes how she was able to rationalise what was happening, keep her emotions in check and manage the whole experience in a very proactive way.

It was the diagnosis of Mae's deafness that presented Ellie with what she describes as a huge crisis. This development impacted on her thoughts and feelings and she found herself reacting to the situation in a way that was not normal for her. Ellie wept and grieved over her daughter's deafness and she has found it incredibly difficult to accept and cope with her daughter's newly diagnosed disability.

Activity

Reflect on your initial thoughts about what was a potential crisis for Ellie.
- How accurate were you in predicting what Ellie would find distressing?
- Would you have had similar responses if this situation happened to you?
- If not, why might that be?

For more information on hydrocephalus and meningitis, visit the Great Ormond Street Hospital website:
www.ich.ucl.ac.uk/gosh_families/information_sheets/hydrocephalus/hydrocephalus_families.html
For more information and support on becoming deaf, the following website offers some useful detail: **http://deaftalk.co.uk/index.htm**

ELIZABETH, JACK AND TIM'S STORY

Elizabeth and Jack are the parents of Tim who, as a small boy, regularly complained of headaches. Tim was referred to a paediatrician who diagnosed childhood migraine and prescribed treatment but, over the next few years, the headaches became progressively worse. Elizabeth sought help for Tim from a variety of alternative and complementary therapists as well as using the prescribed conventional medicine but nothing had any real lasting affect and, at the age of 13, Tim developed a headache that went on to last for months.

Tim was referred back to a paediatrician for further assessment and a brain scan identified an arterial venous malformation (AVM) in the left-hand side of his brain. An AVM is a tangle of blood vessels that have not formed properly and because they result in arterial blood being pumped into small abnormal veins, these smaller vessels are at risk of bursting. It was this pressure that was the cause of Tim's headaches. Tim was referred on to a neurosurgeon, who suggested a non-invasive vascular surgery to plug the malformed vessels and so prevent possible bleeding. Further details about this condition can be found at **www.avmsupport.org.uk**.

A date for surgery was agreed but, ten days before the set date, the AVM in Tim's brain burst, resulting in a massive brain haemorrhage. Tim's mother returned home from work to find her son lying on the living room floor unconscious, in a pool of vomit.

Tim remained unconscious for a week and then underwent a craniotomy (full brain surgery) to remove the blood clot and to restructure the damaged blood vessels. It was a nine-hour operation. Tim recovered from surgery but the family were informed that there could be severe brain damage, personality change, depression and possibly epilepsy. Tim has not shown any sign of severe brain damage, personality change or depression but nine months after surgery he experienced a seizure and three months later he had another. Tim is now adjusting to a life on anti-epileptic drugs.

Activity

This story spans several years during which there appear to be a series of events that could be described as crises. Using your judgement identify, list and provide a short rationale of what you believe to be potential crisis periods.

This exercise is a little more complex as it involves Tim and his parents and each has a unique perspective on what happened, but the potential periods of crisis could be as follows.

The diagnosis of childhood migraine

Elizabeth describes this as being a stressful time. She disliked the thought of Tim being on medication and she searched for alternative and complementary treatments. For Tim headaches were the norm but they did present him with difficulties in functioning. He loved sport but was often unable to play due to his headaches, and computer-based studies always made him feel ill. His teachers were not always sympathetic and Tim regularly made out that he was OK when he clearly was not. Tim's dad had suffered from migraine for years so he accepted the situation as one that everyone just had to put up with.

The diagnosis of the arterial vascular malformation (AVM)

Each person involved had different reactions. Elizabeth had some medical knowledge and the ability to access detailed information on the internet and medical/surgical journals, but what she found increased her anxiety rather than reducing it. Referral to a neurosurgeon confirmed her fears and she describes a sense of dread developing as she contemplated what could happen. Elizabeth struggled with keeping her thoughts and feelings under control and when she was on her own she cried a great deal about what was to come. Tim's father refused to discuss possibilities, taking a very matter-of-fact attitude to the situation and commenting that they should all wait and see. For Tim there was a sense of relief that, at long last, a reason had been found for his headaches and his teachers became much more sympathetic.

The brain haemorrhage

This was the real crisis. Elizabeth knew instantly what had happened when she found Tim semi-conscious on the floor. It was a life-threatening situation that demanded quick decisions and fast action. With the help of her other son she was able to get help and, despite her great anxiety, she was able to brief the paramedics and then hospital staff regarding Tim's condition. This anxiety and images of Tim lying on the floor have returned to trouble Elizabeth on several occasions and she describes an overwhelming sense of panic when Tim is not well, always imagining the worst thing possible.

Elizabeth described how difficult it was to be brave. She knew she needed to let go and weep but felt unable to do so in hospital where she had to be strong and watch over her boy. However, on a short visit home to collect personal items on the second day, she was able to cry and release some of her tension. Her emotional fragility impacted on her relationship with her husband, who was also struggling to deal with his son's situation and unable to support her in the way that she expected. The couple were so traumatised that neither could help the other, which led to further difficulties later on. Tim can only recall a little detail as he drifted in and out of consciousness but he knew he might die and kept the thought in his head that 'I am too young to die'.

For further details on how to recognise and care for people who have experienced brain haemorrhage visit the Stroke Organisation at **www.stroke.org.uk**.

The decision regarding surgery

For Tim's parents the decision regarding surgery had to be made even though it involved more risk. Tim, who was semi-comatose at the point at which the decision was being made, has since stated that he didn't really care what happened to him at that stage and he describes experiencing what he called an epiphany, thinking he had faced death and survived.

The late onset of seizures

This development has resulted in Tim's parents having concerns and anxieties about Tim and his future. Elizabeth describes reliving the fear all over again when Tim first developed seizures. As a family they now have to cope with the reality of Tim's epilepsy, facing their fears and addressing their own and other people's prejudicial ideas about what it is to suffer from seizures.

Tim has to live that experience and cope with the disappointments that his seizures have brought and will bring in future. He had wanted to join the Army but, given his experience and his epilepsy, this is now very unlikely. He uses humour to good effect, making everyone laugh, and he is incredibly proud of his survival. He has enjoyed telling friends of his ordeal and detailing the dramas of his experience and at school he became 'a bit of a legend'. Tim's balanced emotions and his resilience to deal with adversity, alongside a good sense of humour and positive attitude towards life, should enable him to deal with whatever comes his way.

For further detail on coping with epilepsy please visit: **www.epilepsy.org.uk** or telephone 0808 800 5050.

Activity

- What are the similarities in these first two stories?
- To address this you may find it useful to review each story against the detail given in the FRAGILE TEARS model of crisis in Chapter 1 and then compare and contrast the two stories.

Assessing the first two stories

Both of these stories illustrate how the internal factors of self, thoughts and emotions impact on coping skills. The management of these thoughts and emotions led to a series of reasoned actions. Both families were able to give examples of reactions that were understandable at the time of their crisis but that did not have a negative affect on the outcome.

Reviewing the influencing factors detailed in the outer ring of the FRAGILE TEARS crisis model it appears that there are many similarities in these stories. Although there are some differences of age and family situations, both involve a child being seriously ill over a period of time. Periods of illness do not necessarily mean the children were having a crisis and it is important not to over-dramatise stressful periods and create crises where they do not exist. Both of these families were able to be realistic about their child's illness but, when you explore the eventual crisis each family encountered, you can see that both have coped remarkably well.

Key factors in their coping skills involved the support of their family and friends. Having positive caring relationships plays a key role in enabling people to face crisis (Fredrickson *et al.*, 2003). Also, specialised health services and other support agencies were available to them at the time of crisis and neither family blames other people for what happened to their children. Focusing on 'if only' and blaming other people for what goes wrong in our lives is often detrimental and prevents people from moving on. Both families were well educated and informed regarding their child's condition and as service users, treatment plans were always made in agreement with them and not for them. There were some differences in relation to gender. Jack and Tim were very matter-of-fact about the situation and shed no tears but the two women needed to express their emotions and both reported weeping. The adults of both families were professionals with comfortable Western lifestyles and both had sympathetic employers and their income and job were automatically safeguarded. Both families describe the hospital experience as being very uncomfortable but, once back home, their environments were conducive to calm living, providing comfort and security.

The challenge these families now have to face is the disability that their child's illness has left them with. Both families expressed concern about society's attitude towards people who are different and, according to Oliver (1996), disability often leads to marginalisation and discrimination. The families know they will have to adjust their own attitudes and meet the prejudicial ideas of others in the best way that they can to ensure their children are not discriminated against.

The next two stories involve people in relationships that end suddenly.

MONICA'S STORY

Monica had been married to Douglas for 25 years. They had raised two children who had both left home. One day a letter arrived addressed to 'Mr and Mrs X'. It contained a confirmation of a hotel booking for the following weekend. It was a double room. Monica was puzzled. Douglas was going away that weekend with friends to the Isle of Man to watch the TT motorcycle races but the hotel was in Cornwall. She couldn't understand it. She recalls thinking that maybe he had planned a surprise weekend for them but she knew in her heart of hearts that there was something amiss. She waited until he came home and asked him what was going on.

Douglas looked embarrassed and then, as Monica recalls, 'He just came out with it, he was having an affair, and he loved her'. That was all she heard before she flew into a rage. Monica describes how she couldn't believe what she had heard. She demanded that he explain himself and as he tried to tell her he was leaving her she reacted by physically attacking him, hitting him, pulling his hair and screaming at him at the top of her voice. Monica describes the next half hour as mayhem. Douglas went upstairs and collected some personal things: pants, shaving gear, some shirts and a jumper. She pulled at the bag, tearing the shirt he was trying to pack and he pushed her on to the bed. He left the house and did not return for three days.

Monica says that when Douglas returned to the house he probably thought she would be at work but she was there. She hadn't left the house since he had gone. She says she must have looked really unkempt and she couldn't remember exactly what she had done for three days. She cried a great deal and sobbed so loudly that she was surprised the neighbours didn't come round. On the first night she knows she had got very drunk and was very sick the following day. She had broken several things in the house, torn his clothes in the wardrobe, ripped up her wedding photographs and had pulled the telephone out of the socket. Monica describes being shocked at her level of anger and hatred and she had tried to identify other clues that he was having an affair. She wrote down details like 'buying his own pants, changing his aftershave' and she couldn't remember the last time they had made love.

When Douglas found she was in the house he looked upset and she thought for a minute that he had come back: 'Come back to hang his head in shame, to apologise and beg forgiveness' but that was not how it was. He did try to talk to her and he did say he was sorry but he was leaving her. He and his girlfriend had talked about it for months and although he didn't want to make her unhappy he wanted to be with the other woman and not with her.

Douglas then went and told Monica's mother what had happened and he asked her to take care of her. Monica's mother spat at him and told him what he had done was unforgivable and that he would live to regret it. Over the next few weeks, as Monica's rage abated, she became ill. She was so depressed she couldn't get herself out of bed in the mornings, she stopped eating, lost weight and cried a great deal. The GP was called and he prescribed anti-depressants. Douglas had a solicitor write to her asking for a separation and eventual divorce but Monica could not respond as she felt so wretched.

Several months passed and more letters arrived. Douglas wanted a divorce on the grounds of her unreasonable behaviour. 'My unreasonable behaviour; I didn't have the affair!' but Monica felt too tired to contest it. He wanted the family home sold and the proceeds split between the two of them. This was the home they had raised their family in, the home that was her comfort and that was to be lost as well.

Monica is now receiving psychiatric help. She is trying to deal with her depression and the sense of abandonment that her divorce has left her with. The house is on the market and Monica has returned to part-time work. She is slowly building her life back up but this has been a painful experience for Monica that has changed every aspect of her life.

Activity

Monica has encountered difficult life-changing decisions as a result of her husband leaving her. Using the FRAGILE TEARS model, can you identify potential consequences of divorce for men and women?

Reviewing the case study

According to the Office of National Statistics (2008), divorce rates are currently falling and in the year up to August 2008 it is calculated that 11.9 marriages in every 1000 end in divorce. This figure compares with 15 marriages in every 1000 ending in divorce in 2003. Statistics show that while, in general, divorce rates are decreasing the divorce rates are on the increase for couples over 45 years of age.

Activity

Given the statistics regarding divorce rate, what possible explanations could account for this trend?

According to the statistics, infidelity remains the number one reason for seeking divorce, but there is now evidence that financial hardship is resulting in more couples seeking marriage guidance and counselling. For many people divorce is not a financial option. More data on divorces in England and Wales in 2007 are available on the National Statistics website:

www.statistics.gov.uk/statbase/Product.asp?vlnk=14124

The following website offers good advice and supportive detail for those undergoing separation and divorce: **www.helptoheal.co.uk**.

STELLA'S STORY

Stella is a young woman who was raised in what appeared to be a 'normal family'. She is the only girl, she has several brothers and she describes herself to be 'a boy at heart'. Two years ago she found herself to be homeless, thrown out of the family home by her father who she says described her as 'a waste of space and a dirty little tart'. The ejection from her family home came about after a massive row about her being late home after a date with a local boy who was known to the family. The row started on the doorstep when Stella was saying goodnight to her date. The boy was so startled by Stella's father's anger that he mumbled an apology and left quickly. Stella and her father screamed and bawled at each other on the doorstep and, when her mother came to see what was happening, her father slammed the door in Stella's face, refusing her entry and threatening his wife with violence should she attempt to let her in behind his back.

Stella tried to rouse one of her brothers by throwing pebbles at his bedroom window, only to be met by the angry face of her father who threw some of her clothing out of the window and told her to 'get lost and not darken his doorstep again'.

Over the next few days Stella stayed with various friends and sneaked back to her home when her father was out at work. She cried with her mother, who told her that she was too afraid of what her dad might do if she came back. Stella's mother had a black eye and a cut lip. Stella made the decision that to try to get back into the family home would only result in further violence and she made her decision never to go back no matter how hard life became.

Activity

What thoughts and feelings do you think might be experienced by Stella?

Reviewing Stella's story

You may have identified Stella's confusion and her overall feeling of fear caused by her father's angry rejection of her. Stella's thoughts were 'Where would she go, what would she do?' 'Where would she sleep? What had she done?' Her first reaction was to cry and beg her father to let her in. When she realised her father was not going to let her in, her reactions changed; she shouted and screamed obscenities back at her father as he threw her clothes out of the bedroom window.

It may appear that this outburst came out of the blue and could not have been predicted. On the surface this may appear to be a substantial crisis; a young person being rejected from the safety of their own home, but what emerged, as Stella told her story, was that this episode, although a crisis at the time, proved to be a great relief to her and she has detailed how she had been sexually abused by her father for many years. Being refused back into the family home was the end of abuse at her father's hands, and also freed her from the guilt and the anger that she felt when she looked at her mother, who Stella claims 'had not protected her'.

The Centre for Action on Rape and Abuse offers sound advice for people who have experienced rape or abuse and for people who know of someone who needs help at: **www.crcl.org.uk/index.html**, telephone number 01206 769795. Should any person become aware of abuse of children they are required to take action and report their concerns either to the local police, social work department or education authority.

By including Stella's story here it serves as a reminder to us that what appears to be a terrible crisis may become a positive turning point for the person concerned. To offer the reader reassurance, Stella did eventually find accommodation and she has received professional counselling regarding her father's abuse, but it took her a long time to agree to see anyone other than people who could give her direct help with coping with being homeless.

Stella described how annoying it has been for her that almost everyone she came into contact with wanted to know why her father threw her out. All the 'helping agencies' she came into contact with when she was looking for somewhere to stay asked her for an explanation or reason for her father throwing her out. She lost her job and had difficulty in claiming benefits, mainly because she would be abusive towards the people who had to interview her. She was accused of making herself homeless and did not receive much sympathy until she came into contact with a charitable organisation that provided her with a bed and then helped her to reorganise her life.

Stella is now 'on the up' and she has set herself ordinary goals – 'get a place of my own, maybe get a bloke' – but her crisis has turned her life around. She is free from an abusive relationship but still has a long way to go to achieve her goals.

According to Centre Point in London, 45 per cent of young people who become homeless do so as a consequence of family violence and abuse. According to the Children's Society, some of the children who run away from home are only eight years old. (**www.childrenssociety.org. uk**). Statistics are vague on how many young people are homeless at any one time but interesting details are available at **www.centrepoint.org.uk**, telephone number 0845 466 3400, along with other web links to valid sources of information and support.

According to Homeless Link, the national membership organisation for homelessness agencies in England, ethnic minorities are particularly vulnerable to homelessness. Reasons for this are said to include 'deprivation, social exclusion caused by poverty, unemployment, low educational achievements, overcrowding, stress, ill-health and social isolation, etc.', which are said to affect 'a greater proportion of ethnic minority individuals than white people'. Sources and further details available at:

www.homeless.org.uk/policyandinfo/issues/youngpeople
telephone number 020 7960 3010.

Activity

Stella refused help in the initial stages. Have you ever attempted to help anyone who has refused your offer of help?
- How did you address that and what was the outcome for you and the person you wanted to help?
- What can you learn from this situation?

Many people refuse help in crisis situations and it could be argued that their lives may deteriorate even further as a result of not asking for or refusing help when it is offered to them. Many people are not aware of the help available to them and, as a helper, perhaps your biggest strength lies in knowing how to go about searching for appropriate help. Each person has to be viewed as a unique individual and, as helpers, we need to step back from imposing our own agenda on to those who appear to need help. It is important to recognise that people in crisis are often not in control of their thoughts and feelings and may react inappropriately. This may result in you receiving the impact of their distress – for example, being shouted out or verbally abused. The current campaign of 'zero tolerance' of verbal or physical abuse towards people who are working in the public sector needs to be applied carefully. We do need to give consideration to those who are clearly distressed. Time out, asking people to come back later or working through an intermediary are all strategies that we can use to ensure that people are safe and that appropriate care is offered.

The next three stories all involve illness in adulthood.

MARTIN'S STORY

Martin's wife was the first person to notice he had a lump in his neck. He had been aware that there was something there and he also had a patch of dry skin. There were jokes made about skin cancer and Martin had an appointment to see his GP and asked her to take a look. A blood test was ordered along with a prescription of steroid cream for the dry patch and a referral was made for him to see an Ear Nose and Throat (ENT) specialist.

The appointment with the specialist clashed with a first day in a new job so Martin cancelled, but he did go back to the GP for the results of the blood test, which revealed a raised white blood cell count that is usually indicative of something being amiss. The GP mentioned lymphoma and told him he must go and see the specialist. Martin kept the next appointment and noticed that the nurse who was with the doctor during the consultation wore a badge that said 'Macmillan Nurse'.

Martin underwent tests and a scan and described his reaction to what the consultant said as 'It is all a bit of a blur . . . at first it does not sink in . . . he said there is a cancerous lump, a number of masses there, he said this is serious.' Martin described how he couldn't believe this was really happening and then, in a moment of realisation, he asked the question 'is this going to kill me then?' Martin took the doctor's hesitation to indicate that it might and he sat through an explanation of what was to happen, including surgery and chemotherapy, without fully taking the information in.

Activity

What are the potential fears and anxieties of people who are newly diagnosed with cancer?

Reviewing Martin's story

This is how Martin described his fears and anxieties. 'Fear of the unknown things that are going to happen to me, fear of cancer, people die from cancer and, before they die, they have a bad time with the chemotherapy, their hair falls out, you feel lousy and spend a lot of time with your head down the toilet. I can't do this, other people can do this but I am not strong enough.'

Martin is now in a position where he can joke about having cancer. Members of his family are in the medical profession so they are able to help explain conversations with consultants and treatment plans, and they helped to prepare Martin for how tough treatment was going to be and how best he could manage it. He clearly identifies that being told he had cancer was the worst part of his crisis. Since then he has become used to discussing his cancer and talking about his symptoms, what is helpful and what has been difficult. He trusts the doctors and nurses, literally with his life, and takes comfort in their efficiency, careful checking and knowing who he is. The nurses talk to him about his health, his family, their family and everyday life in general.

Martin has been surprised at how well his family have accepted his illness. His children accepted that daddy needed to go to hospital and his daughter hugs him regularly, checks if he is feeling better and, when he lost his hair, she said 'daddy you have lost your hair you silly daddy'. That makes Martin laugh and he has shared that once you get into the practicalities of it happening you then get on and deal with it.

Like many people who are given this diagnosis, Martin described how he has searched for reasons for his cancer and once, when with friends who were smoking, he felt a deep anger. He had never smoked but he is the one with the cancer, a fit, healthy young man who has always looked after himself, never done anyone a bad turn, but bad things happen to good people and Martin knows that no one is really to blame. He now wants to focus on his emotions and pays attention to his diet. As a teacher he has a protected job while he is ill and sick pay keeps his family together. No one knows what the future holds for him and facing this crisis is the hardest thing he has ever done.

Cancer Help UK is the patient information website of Cancer Research UK and their web pages serve as a valuable resource to patients and professionals alike, but their site comes with a firm reminder that if you are in any way worried that you may have cancer you should go to see your GP.

www.cancerhelp.org.uk/default.asp

ZENA AND ALEX'S STORY

Zena and Alex are in their 40s and newly married. One morning Zena noticed that her big toe on her left foot had become sore and looked discoloured. Being a diabetic, she recognised this as a danger sign that required urgent attention. Over the next few months, she first lost her toe, then her lower leg, finishing with a mid-thigh amputation.

For further information on diabetes please visit the following website: **www.diabetes.org.uk**.

Zena described her thoughts and feelings when facing amputation and her main concerns were for her new husband: 'he didn't want to marry a cripple, it's too much for him to cope with'. Like many people in crisis she describes looking for reasons as to why this should happen to her. She doesn't drink, doesn't smoke and describes herself as a reasonable person but some of her thoughts scare her. There have been times when she has wanted to die, when she has had enough and when she thinks she cannot do this anymore.

Zena described how she has had to battle with high levels of anxiety. She had a phobia of hospitals, acquired in childhood, which has been reinforced by subsequent events, including the death of one of her daughters from a previous marriage. In the initial stages of her gangrene Zena was given a choice of having her toe amputated or having further antibiotic treatment and she opted for amputation knowing that antibiotics were not guaranteed to work. The doctor asked her if she 'wanted time to grieve for the toe'. Zena replied she did not, as the death of one of her daughters was grief enough, but she wonders if this was the reason for getting an emergency visit at home from a psychiatric nurse. Although she was initially angry about the suggestion of her 'being of unsound mind', she is now able to laugh about it and appreciates her doctor's anxiety about her mental health.

Zena knew she had to have her leg amputated, but at times she wished she had died. She not only feared reduced mobility, but also 'not being useful or needed'. Being in pain was not a new experience, but she had not anticipated the pain from using her arms to get up and down stairs, pain in her hips from the uneven leg or overuse of her 'good' leg. At the start of the amputations, all she wanted was to be safe at home with her husband and her cats. She took her own pillows into hospital and coped with the episodes of panic by repeating to herself: 'This is shit, but I can win, I know what's best for me.' Reading, listening to music, visits from friends and the continued support of her husband kept her going.

Zena felt and still feels guilt that she has become less of a wife and more of a burden to her husband. Having only one leg restricts what she can do and throughout this experience the levels of pain have varied. The combination of pain, analgesia and other medication affected her short-term memory and her sense of time, and Zena recalls frustration and fear when she could not remember if things had been done.

Prior to all this Zena had experience of disability as a result of bringing up and supporting her daughter, who was severely disabled. She was aware of what various agencies had to offer and she wanted to get herself as independent as possible as soon as possible, both from the point of view of maintaining her physical ability but also, as she knew from previous episodes of ill health, that being immobile could possibly lead to depression.

Zena describes how the internet provided her with a great deal of information about aids for mobility and personal hygiene. When her first artificial limb arrived, Zena was determined to use it as best she could and she practised moving and walking and, despite the leg being too big for her, she persevered. Zena has now started to ride and swim again, and is able to drive herself around in her new adapted car.

With regard to the helping agencies, Zena commented that professional denial of her problems was a major cause of stress and there were times when she 'felt ignored or made to feel small'. On one occasion she asked if she could have an automatic light installed outside the front door so she could see up the step to get in her house. She was asked 'Why would you want to go out alone in the dark?', as if a grown woman with a wooden leg wouldn't want to be out in the dark.

Activity

People who are in helping positions can inadvertently be patronising, making judgements about what other people should or should not be doing. Have you any experience of this? How did the person respond? How might patronising someone affect the helping relationship?

NHS Choices, available at: **www.nhs.uk/Livewell/Disability**, contains really useful information about adjusting to life with a disability.

ROSE AND SPIKE'S STORY

Spike was riding his motor bike when a car turned into his path from a side road. The impact somersaulted Spike over the car, he had multiple internal injuries and was taken to intensive care in an air ambulance. Rose was at work when her son and a policewoman arrived to tell her the news. Spike had serious injuries and had been taken to a regional intensive care unit and she likens receiving this news to being hit with a heavy weight. She reacted by thinking 'I must keep it together, sort things out and stay in charge' and this thinking was accompanied with a burst of energy that carried her over the next few days.

Rose stayed at the hospital, but hardly slept and she describes reacting to nursing and medical staff in a very precise, matter-of-fact way. She described a sense of guilt that she functioned at a high level when under pressure. She recalled she was the same when diagnosed with cancer. She went home, organised work and family and then took herself off for surgery. Keeping active and being efficient was Rose's way of coping and she saved her tears for when she had the privacy to cry out loud.

The extended family rallied round, working out a rota for visiting and giving Rose a break. When Spike came home, they continued to visit and to offer their support, and Rose recalls that she felt as if she was running a B&B but recognised that family members had a need to help as they struggled to cope with the outcome of Spike's injuries. Rose describes how her daughter, a nurse for people with learning disabilities, was able to make really useful suggestions in respect of behavioural approaches and for ways of stimulating Spike to extend his cognitive function. However, Rose found herself wishing she could have some peace from family members and some time on her own and this created ambivalent feelings that she then had to cope with too.

Outside the family, various agencies were helpful. The internet proved a valuable source of information but Rose describes the claim for compensation as a traumatic experience. 'My life was invaded by it, because Spike had multiple serious injuries, he had to see a lot of expert witnesses from both sides of the case. He had 28 different assessments, in different locations, all across the country.' Spike became more and more irritable with meeting new people and being repeatedly 'tested', as he viewed it. Rose suggested that some 'experts' treated them as if they were stupid and they were patronising, and it seemed to the couple that others were just out to make money.

Assessment at home would have provided a better picture of Spike's needs and Rose describes how, after each assessment, she had to write a report or a response. She did this in the evening after a day of caring and probably driving around the country and describes how she felt:

> I got 'claim fatigue'; I can understand how people get worn down and settle or give up. I kept going because of a sense of justice. Spike was not to blame, and we didn't harbour any ill feeling toward the man who did it, it was just an accident. But, the more assessments and reports, the more I thought this was just a game for the solicitors and sheer bloody-mindedness kept me from caving in.

Rose gave up work to care for Spike and ending a long and successful career so abruptly was a significant loss for her but she wanted to 'be with him, care for him, be at his side'. She can see that Spike still has frequent episodes of pain, as the nerve and blood supplies were torn out of his shoulder. He has difficulty with breathing due to restricted lung capacity and a damaged diaphragm. Sometimes he becomes tearful when watching TV, sobbing uncontrollably, but he cannot explain fully what has caused the emotional reaction, he just says 'it's sad'. Rose wonders if he has some trauma memories, not of the accident, but from later events during his recovery. 'Maybe he can't explain because he can't find the words, or maybe he's a man who can't explain how he feels.'

Fortunately Rose and Spike had enough money saved to cope with the unexpected costs of travelling to appointments, adapting the house and other costs. They both have a pension and some investments and they can just manage but Rose fears for the future and what it might bring. Having had this major crisis she knows that others may follow and she fears becoming less able to cope. The couple may have to move and are considering moving to an adapted bungalow, and that in itself will be stressful for both of them.

Activity

When a crisis such as this happens it has a deep impact on others involved, particularly loved ones who give up their job to become full-time carers. How might that change in circumstance affect people like Rose?

Useful websites and contacts

Caring for a loved one who is physically disabled can be exhausting and there are many support groups and agencies that offer practical help as well as psychological support and information. The following web address is for the Help and Care Organisation, which is a registered charity offering practical advice and valuable links for carers. **www.helpandcare. org.uk/home.aspx**, telephone number 0300 111 3303.

When a person is incapacitated following an accident, the impact on their income and their future lives can result in further hardship for them and their family. In most cases of personal injury there is a right to claim compensation. For straightforward advice as to how to make a claim for personal injury visit the Citizens Advice Bureau available online at: **www.adviceguide.org.uk/index/your_rights/legal_system/ personal_injuries.htm**

The following story involves a financial crisis, imprisonment and how a family have tried to cope.

BOB AND GILL'S STORY

Bob is a 42-year-old married man, with three daughters. Six years ago, he served an 18-month jail sentence for fraud. He was found guilty of 'siphoning off' payments made to his office and paying them into an account opened by another man in his office. They and one other person then split the money three ways. Bob recalls that he did not feel as though he was 'really' a criminal as other people did much worse things. He wanted the money as he was getting into debt with his mortgage and other bills.

He knew there was something wrong when he went to work, but was not allowed in until he was interviewed by the police. The next day, he was charged with fraud and arrested. He was found guilty and, at his trial, the judge said 'Your sentence may seem lenient, but that reflects my belief that you are naïve and easily led, rather than deliberately criminally minded.'

Activity

Bob's partner Gill comments that the whole family were sentenced when Bob was found guilty and sent down. What might be the effect on family members when a crisis such as this happens?

Reviewing Bob and Gill's story

Gill describes how people she knew would 'go out of their way to avoid passing me on the street'. She says the girls were bullied at school and the story was splashed all over the local newspaper so everyone around her knew. Shortly after Bob's arrest, Gill learned the extent of their debt. Credit cards, bank loans and mortgage arrears had all been hidden from her. Bob had managed all those things while she just managed the kids. They always went shopping together and he had never indicated that they couldn't afford anything. She had thought everything to be OK.

The house was eventually repossessed by the building society and the family found themselves having to move into a two-bedroomed flat living off state benefits. This provided some relief for Gill as relocating meant that her new neighbours did not know who they were. The girls changed school but Gill lived in fear of them and of herself being recognised. Credit card bills were frozen via a debt relief order and eventually wiped clean but both Gill and Bob now have no credit rating. Given the current financial regulations it is unlikely that they will be able to get credit again for a long time.

Gill described how she got through the 18 months by putting Bob into a separate mental compartment. Her father was very supportive. Gill describes him as her rock and although her mother has helped out too, her opinion of Bob is very low because, as Gill says, 'she has to live with the shame as well'. She admits many mood changes and, after the initial shock of what Bob had done and him being sent to prison wore off, she found she hated and loved him at the same time, 'like turning a switch on and off'. She still finds it incomprehensible that he did it, saying 'he is such a quiet reliable man and he is so good with the kids but now he is a criminal'.

Once Bob was released from open prison Gill was able to get herself back into full-time work and although it doesn't pay particularly well there is regular overtime. Bob stays at home, he cooks and cleans and takes care of the children but he is fearful that he will never get another job again. His applications for jobs are half-hearted as his expectation is to be rejected despite lots of reassurance from his probation officer.

For information regarding help with managing debt visit the Citizens Advice Bureau **www.citizensadvice.org.uk/index.htm**, or contact the National Debt line for free and confidential advice, **www.nationaldebtline. co.uk**, or telephone 0808 808 4000.

For advice on bullying, contact Childline on 0800 11 11 or visit their website **www.childline.org.uk**

For a support organisation for families who have a relative in prison, visit **www.prisonersfamilieshelpline.org.uk** or telephone 0808 808 2003.

The one thing we can be sure of is that some day we will die. When we are the ones left behind we need to adjust to new ways of living. The next three stories are about people coping with grief.

KATE'S STORY

Kate was at work when she received a phone call telling her to come home quickly. She describes a feeling of dread and instantly deduced that it was about her father, but she was able to stay calm enough to drive home. There were two ambulances and Kate ran into the house to find her dad lying on the kitchen floor, surrounded by paramedics trying to resuscitate him.

Kate describes how the living room was chaos, with her two-year-old daughter crying and her mother hysterical. A neighbour stepped in to help and took the little girl in her arms while Kate tried to calm her mum. The paramedics worked on Kate's father for another 45 minutes, but he did not recover.

Kate recalls that, despite having an overwhelming sense of panic – she says she 'couldn't breathe' – that she knew she had to 'take charge, had to cope'. Losing her dad was the worst thing to happen but she needed to make sure the rest of her family were safe and she had to deal with the officials. She described her thoughts as being confused but she was still able to rationalise what had to be done. She asked one of the paramedics to get her dad a quilt to wrap him in, to keep him warm. She knew he was dead but this action meant that she could sit on the floor with him and cuddle him until his body was removed from the house. This simple action, Kate believes, helped her cope and recalling that action brings her comfort even now.

The memory of her dad's death is still very real for Kate. She recalls being numb, cold and having to cope with her panic. She felt she was 'in a glass bubble', which seemed to isolate her from the rest of the world for weeks after her father's death. She could not sleep, so was prescribed night sedation by her GP. Despite being desperate to rest she carried on caring for her children and looking after her mum.

For the next three years Kate went into overdrive. She didn't sleep well, skipped meals and ignored the stomach pain, which eventually resulted in her emergency admission to hospital due to peritonitis. Being told she was very seriously ill forced Kate to re-evaluate her life. She had feared for her own mental health and thought she was going mad with grief but, with the support of friends and work colleagues, she is now able to focus on the most important things, her family and her health. She expresses a deep gratitude to those who have helped her: the emergency services, the GP, the mental health services for help with her mum, and she used the Samaritans and CRUSE in the early days following her father's death. For details on those two organisations please use the following web and telephone links:

www.samaritans.org.uk 08357 90 90 90 and
www.crusebereavementcare.org.uk

Activity

Experiencing the sudden death of a loved one may result in a variety of responses. Using the inner circle of the FRAGILE TEARS model, identify common responses to sudden death.

For further detail and support regarding common experiences following death visit the Royal College of Psychiatrists web pages at: **www.rcpsych. ac.uk/mentalhealthinfoforall/problems/bereavement/bereavement.aspx** or telephone the Bereavement and Advice Centre on 0800 634 9494.

LUKE'S STORY

Luke and his wife had been looking forward to the birth of their baby, who they already knew from a previous scan was a little girl. The baby had been carried for her full term and nothing had been a cause for concern during the pregnancy. On the day that labour commenced Luke happily took his wife and her overnight bag to hospital and the little girl was born shortly after. The baby did not survive the day.

Luke describes his newly-born daughter as being 'shuffled off' into a corner of the delivery room, where the staff used equipment on her. He describes the baby as being very quiet, not crying, but making small whimpering noises. Luke recalls hearing one member of staff saying 'She's going off', which he thought was an odd thing to say but he now knows what they meant.

The baby was taken for emergency care to the special care baby unit (SCBU); Luke went with her initially but then he returned to be with his wife. They waited for any news together, both of them realising how serious the situation was and fearing the worst for their baby. A doctor eventually came to tell them that their daughter was seriously ill and could not survive. He asked if they wanted to see her and he arranged for them to see and hold their dying baby until she was gone. They left the hospital for home and Luke describes a sense of dislocation from reality and expectation, 'Three hours after having a baby, my wife walked out of the hospital with the bag she brought in – but without her baby, and we went home.' Luke went back to work the next day. The following week the funeral took place in the hospital chapel with close family and friends only and the baby was then cremated.

Luke chose to end his story there. The death of his daughter was over a decade ago and he expresses a need to look forward and not back. He sought no help with his grief, quietly dealing with his own thoughts and feelings so as not to impose any demands on his wife. They made a decision to normalise life as quickly as possible but each year on the day of her birth the family mark the occasion to remember her.

Activity

According to Lovell (1997, cited in Payne *et al.*,1999), miscarriage, still birth and neonatal death have not always been acknowledged by society but the loss of a baby is now considered by some to be the most poignant loss of all. What is your view?

Before the twentieth century neonate and infant death was not unusual but, with medical advancement and societal changes, we are usually now able to successfully rear our young to adulthood and the death of a neonate is now relatively rare in our society. However, the grief that follows a neonate death can be very painful because as well as losing the baby, the parents also lose the dreams, hopes and aspirations that they had for their baby. For further information and support on the death of a neonate the Still Birth and Neonatal Death Society (SANDS) is a valuable support agency for people in this situation. Contact by telephone number 020 7436 5881 or online at **www.uk-sands.org**

DOROTHY'S STORY

Dorothy was married with two children and her family was struck by tragedy in 1969 when, following a day trip out, their car was hit by a large bus. Dorothy's husband was badly injured with a fractured skull and her nine-year-old son was also seriously hurt. Dorothy's husband was in a coma for four days and then drifted in and out of consciousness over the next week or so. She stayed by his side for as long as she could, leaving him only to go and see her son who was being treated in another hospital. Sadly her son lost his fight for life and he died in hospital. Dorothy had to arrange her son's funeral while her husband was still in hospital suffering from the consequences of severe head injury. Despite his disabilities she insisted upon taking him home as quickly as she could, nursing him through his rehabilitation period and helping him with every aspect of daily living. The couple tried to get back to normal living but another tragedy hit them when their daughter was also killed in a road traffic accident.

If this was not enough for a family to bear, Dorothy's husband then went on to develop Alzheimer's disease and he needed love, care and constant supervision until his recent death. Dorothy reflects back upon her life and the losses she has experienced – both her children and then coping with losing her husband to dementia. It appears that she has had more crises than any other person we interviewed and yet she presents as a strong person who finds comfort in her Christian faith. She hopes that she will see her loved ones again one day but Dorothy's mother-in-law, who was a regular churchgoer, stopped going to church after the death of her grandson.

People react differently to loss. For some people faith becomes a great support at times of loss but for others faith too is lost as a result of death.

Activity

What religious faiths are you aware of and how can those faiths be helpful to people in dealing with death, dying, grief and mourning?

Reviewing Dorothy's story

Religion, regardless of faith, provides people with an understanding of the world and religious customs inform people how to behave, particularly at the time of death and in the period of mourning. In today's society, where living our lives in accordance with our religious beliefs is said to be decreasing, it is becoming more commonplace to talk about spirituality and our personal search for meaning. Neuberger (1994) offers detailed guidance on how to care for dying people of different faiths and Cooke (2000) provides a practical guide to holistic care at the end of life. For detail regarding death customs and rituals across different faiths and cultures visit:

http://dying.about.com/od/cultureanddeath/Cultural_Perspectives_on_Death_Dying_and_Bereavement.htm

The following website offers a range of advice and useful strategies that can be used to help people cope with grief. It takes a practical approach to a complex problem that affects or will affect us all at some point in our lives. **www.bbc.co.uk/relationships/coping_with_grief**. Finally, Currer (2001) and Sutcliffe *et al.* (1998) provide valuable detail about the carer's/helper's role in working with the dying and the bereaved.

SUMMARY

In this chapter we have shared people's stories, offered exercises designed to facilitate an empathic approach and provided a range of resources we trust that you will find useful. We list those resources again here and Chapter 3 will take you through theoretical perspectives on crisis and individual responses to it.

SUPPORT AGENCIES AND RESOURCES FOR PEOPLE IN CRISIS

Great Ormond Street Hospital for Children NHS Trust (GOSH) and UCL Institute of Child Health (ICH). Available at: **www.ich.ucl.ac.uk/gosh_families/information_sheets/ hydrocephalus/hydrocephalus_families.html**

Cryer P. (2008) Deaf talk. Available at: **http://deaftalk.co.uk/index.htm**

Arterial Venous Malformation Support. Available at: **www.avmsupport.org.uk**

The Stroke Association. Available at: **www.stroke.org.uk**

Epilepsy Action Group. Available at: **www.epilepsy.org.uk**

National Statistics Office (Online). Available at: **www.statistics.gov.uk/statbase/Product.asp?vlnk=14124**

Help To Heal Counselling Services (Online). Available at: **www.helptoheal.co.uk**

Centre for Action on Rape and Abuse. Available at: **www.crcl.org.uk/index.html**

The Children's Society. Available at: **www.childrenssociety.org.uk**

Centre Point Organisation. Giving Homeless Young People a Future. Available at: **www.centrepoint.org.uk**

Homeless Link. Frontline Agencies in Partnership. Available at: **www.homeless.org.uk/policyandinfo/issues/youngpeople**

Cancer Research UK. Available at: **www.cancerhelp.org.uk/default.asp**

Diabetes UK. Available at: **www.diabetes.org.uk**

NHS Choices. Available at: **www.nhs.uk/Livewell/Disability**

Citizens Advice Bureau. Available at: **www.adviceguide.org.uk/index/ your_rights/legal_system/personal_injuries.htm**

bbc.co.uk Health Pages. Relationships and coping with grief. Available at: **www.bbc.co.uk/relationships/coping_with_grief**

Help and Care Organisation UK. Available at: **www.helpandcare.org.uk/home.aspx**

The Samaritans Organisation UK. Available at: **www.samaritans.org.uk**

CRUSE Bereavement Care (Online) Available at: **www.crusebereavementcare.org.uk**

Royal College of Psychiatrists. Available at: **www.rcpsych.ac.uk/ mentalhealthinfoforall/problems/bereavement/bereavement.aspx**

Still Birth and Neonatal Death Society (SANDS) (online) Available at **www.uk-sands.org**

http://dying.about.com/od/cultureanddeath/Cultural_Perspectives_ on_Death_Dying_and_Bereavement.htm

REFERENCES

Cooke, H. (2000) *When Someone Dies*. Oxford: Butterworth Heinemann

Currer, C. (2001) *Responding to Grief. Dying, Bereavement and Social Care*. London: Palgrave Press

Fredrickson, B., Tugade, M., Waugh, C. and Larkin, G. (2003) 'What good are positive emotions in crises?' *Journal of Personality and Social Psychology*. Available at: **www-psych.stanford.edu**

Office of National Statistics (2008) **www.statistics.gov.uk/statbase/ Product.asp?vlnk=14124**

Oliver, M. (1996) *Understanding Disability*. Basingstoke: Macmillan

Neuberger, J. (1994) *Caring for People of Different Faiths*. London: Mosby

Payne, S., Horn, S. and Relf, M. (1999) *Loss and Bereavement*. Milton Keynes: Open University Press

Sutcliffe, P., Tufnell, G. and Cornish, U. (eds) (1998) *Working with the Dying and Bereaved: Systemic Approaches to Therapeutic Work*. Basingstoke: Macmillan

Chapter 3

Crisis: Theoretical perspectives

Key themes

This chapter introduces you to:

- crisis theory: schools of thought;
- the physiology of crisis: a neurobiological approach;
- behavioural applications in the understanding of crisis;
- a cognitive approach to understanding crisis;
- the psychoanalytical theory of crisis;
- using transactional analysis to explain crisis;
- grief theory;
- a humanistic perspective.

AN INTRODUCTION TO CRISIS THEORY

Crisis theory has its origins in psychology. As a discipline psychology seeks to observe, explain, understand and predict human behaviour. Within psychology there are schools of thought that focus on different aspects of mind and behaviour, and each one offers a perspective on the behaviour being studied. Within each school of thought there is a range of theories and we are going to explore some of the key theories that offer explanations of what happens to us when we experience personal crises.

People experience crises and critical life events throughout their lives; some experience more than others and, in the Western world, emotional distress and psychological discomfort are considered to be inevitable following a personal crisis. It is important to note that the concept of being an autonomous person and being able to control one's own destiny is very much a Western ideal. People from other parts of the world have other principles and, for many, behaviour and ways of living are determined by their cultural heritage and religious background. This is an important concept as it goes some way to explain why people respond to crisis in different ways.

In Chapter 1 we offered our definition of crisis as: 'an unexpected, serious, usually short-term event that presents us with a range of emotional thoughts and feelings that impact upon our behaviour and upon our relationships with ourselves and others'. The discussion in Chapter 1 led us to establish that crisis is often unexpected and impacts on people in different ways but what is common is that crisis demands that decisions need to be made and something needs to change in response to the crisis.

When people attempt to deal with crisis they often resort to long-held coping strategies and this was illustrated by some of the case studies outlined in Chapter 2. Indeed, it can be argued that, on occasions, it is because our previously used coping strategies and behaviours don't work that we find ourselves experiencing personal crisis.

There are several recognised theories that attempt to explain why we have different reactions to life events, and why life events become a crisis resulting in mental distress for some but not for others. This chapter will explain several theories about this, with emphasis on the aspects that are particularly concerned with understanding crisis and trauma, including: neurobiological and physiological aspects, behavioural and cognitive approaches, psychoanalytic theories, transactional analysis and humanistic theories.

PHYSIOLOGICAL EXPLANATIONS AND THE NEUROBIOLOGICAL APPROACH

The neurobiological approach in psychology focuses on what happens in the body when we experience stress. When we perceive ourselves to be in danger there is an automatic physiological reaction most commonly called the 'fight or flight reaction', and sometimes referred to as 'fight, flight or freeze reaction'. You can see this reaction very clearly in the animal kingdom when, for example, a cat unexpectedly sees a dog.

Activity

What would you expect to see if a local cat unexpectedly met up with a dog on the street?

It is likely that your response will include some if not all of the following. The cat would immediately raise its height to look scarier by arching its back and standing on its toes. Its fur would stand on end and it would pull its facial muscles back as far as possible to emit a terrifying hiss and show an alarming set of teeth. With claws exposed, the cat may possibly 'freeze' in this position in its terror and this may, in turn, be sufficient to frighten the dog away. Alternatively, the cat could quickly lash out with its claws, catching the dog off guard and, in the ensuing 'fight', the dog may come off worse for wear, though remember that cat and dog fights are not always predictable. The other option for the cat is to take flight and run off at great speed. This theory of the fight, flight or freeze reaction has its origins in the work of Walter Cannon in the late 1920s and it has become the cornerstone of physiological explanations of how we deal with and respond to fear.

While this reaction may be useful on some occasions for human beings as a response to fear, fighting or running away is not always the best thing to do when faced with fearful or anxiety-provoking situations.

Activity

- Can you identify some possible situations in which it might be beneficial for us to fight or run away?
- Can you now identify situations in which it would be inappropriate to attempt to fight or run away?

Perhaps you were able to identify some experiences of your own. For the purpose of illustration, imagine what you would do if a bomb went off in your locality. It is likely that you would experience a physiological rush of energy and it would be appropriate for you to run for cover. If you were faced with an aggressor who was clearly going to attempt to harm you, that rush of energy might enable you to fight your way out of danger. However, if your fear is a perceived fear rather than a direct danger to your physical safety such as, for example, fear of failing your next exam, it would not be appropriate to fight your way out of the examination room or run for the hills.

Understanding what happens to our bodies during the fight or flight reaction can be helpful in enabling us to learn how to deal with and control some of the physiological responses that take place during crisis situations. Figure 1 identifies what happens to us when we are exposed to fear.

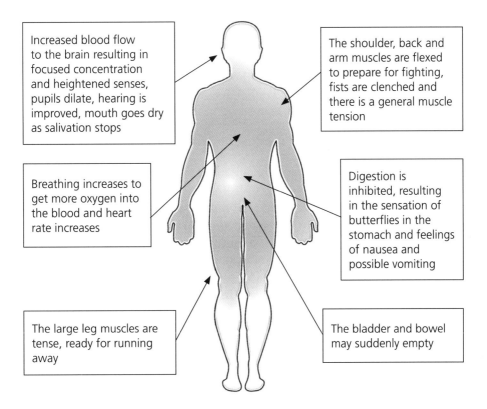

Increased blood flow to the brain resulting in focused concentration and heightened senses, pupils dilate, hearing is improved, mouth goes dry as salivation stops

The shoulder, back and arm muscles are flexed to prepare for fighting, fists are clenched and there is a general muscle tension

Breathing increases to get more oxygen into the blood and heart rate increases

Digestion is inhibited, resulting in the sensation of butterflies in the stomach and feelings of nausea and possible vomiting

The large leg muscles are tense, ready for running away

The bladder and bowel may suddenly empty

Figure 1 Physiological responses to fear

The autonomic nervous system

This physiological response to fear is triggered by our autonomic nervous system, with our brain sending out messages all over the body via our nervous and endocrine systems. These messages influence every living cell within our body, controlling every action and reaction to change. Some of these actions are under our voluntary control, such as choosing to pick up a book, and other actions are involuntary in that they happen without you thinking about it.

Breathing

Breathing can be viewed as an involuntary action because, most of the time, we don't even realise we are doing it. Our breathing speeds up and slows down as it reacts to the demands of the body for oxygen, so we pant during and after exercise and our breathing slows down when we are relaxed or asleep. When we are anxious we may overbreathe by breathing too rapidly or too deeply. This is called hyperventilation, which is breathing in excess of what the body needs and results in the body having too much oxygen and too little carbon dioxide in the blood. Although considered an involuntary action, breathing can be brought under our voluntary control by, for example, practising slow breathing to calm us down. This ability to control some of our actions and reactions will be explored later when we look at helping people cope with crisis but a basic understanding of how the autonomic nervous system works will enable you to understand what happens during the physiological response to fear, stress and anxiety.

Achieving balance

The autonomic nervous system consists of two parts: the sympathetic nervous system, which is responsible for the physiological response to stress, and the parasympathetic nervous system, which acts to bring the body back to normality or back into balance. The maintenance of this balance within the body is sometimes referred to as maintaining homeostasis. The sympathetic nervous system comes into action when danger is perceived and some of the results of the sympathetic nervous system being activated are detailed in Figure 1, illustrating the body preparing to defend itself in times of danger: we become focused on the danger, our senses intensify, our heart and breathing rate increases, our digestion is interrupted and our muscles tense up for action as we prepare for fight or flight.

This physiological reaction serves a very useful purpose in preparing us to defend ourselves and keep us safe in times of danger, but it can be detrimental to our health if it occurs repeatedly over a period of time, particularly when it occurs as a response to psychological stress rather than imminent danger. As human beings we worry, get anxious and 'stressed out' about mortgages, recession, relationships, children, parents, our jobs, our education and a whole host of other things. This is what sets us aside from most animals, the majority of which are only concerned with basic survival. Our problem is that worry or stressing out over these aspects in our lives turns on that physiological response. Overexposure to that physiological response can result in long-term health problems. High blood pressure, heart disease, vascular disorders, neck and shoulder problems, back problems, long-term digestive problems, hormonal disorders, diabetes, cancer, generalised anxiety disorders, hair loss, sexual dysfunction and psychological difficulties have all been associated with chronic stress.

Gibson (2006) explains the continuum of psychological rehabilitation following a crisis and identifies four broad stages of shock, realisation, acknowledgement and adaptation. She claims that this process may include periods of regression as well as progression, acknowledging that some people 'fight the chaos while some will flight the realities of the situation with reactions that include psychological withdrawal associated with denial' (Gibson, 2006, p. 37).

To find out more about the physiology of stress and its impact upon our health, visit **www.working-well.org/articles/pdf/Stress1.pdf**, where you will find useful articles and links to relevant research, as well as an overview of the stress hormones and biological reactions.

Applying neurobiological explanations

In the personal narratives summarised in Chapter 2 we examined individual accounts of their thoughts, feelings, actions and reactions for evidence of the physiological response. Elizabeth discussed the sense of panic that she experienced on discovering her son unconscious and how her thoughts and feelings became very focused on keeping Tim and herself safe. She suggested that her intense fear was transferred into what she called a 'protective fierceness' and that she reacted to situations without thought and sometimes with an aggressive overtone. When Tim was in hospital she watched over him constantly, ready to tackle any member of staff who she believed was not acting in accordance with the care that Tim should receive. She described how she 'lived on her nerves', managing with only snippets of sleep, while watching her son and the staff with an intensity that she had never experienced before. Her stomach was upset and she found it difficult to eat. Over a period of two weeks she lost weight and by the time Tim was discharged home she was exhausted.

Ellie describes her feelings and thoughts when Mae was diagnosed as profoundly deaf and she says that she felt completely isolated and alone and was feeling very scared and emotionally numb. She talked about how she tried not to be frightened, by trying to take control of her thoughts, but found that she focused on negative thoughts such as things that she may have done wrong and what the medics might have done wrong. The negative thoughts led Ellie to a deep anger that was difficult for her to contain and, with heart racing and trembling hands, she called her GP with the intention of screaming at her for what she perceived as being her mistake. Fortunately, by the time the GP came to the phone, Ellie had regained her control but that anger remained a problem for her long after the event.

Martin described how he had reacted to the diagnosis of his cancer, saying that although he was aware he was in the clinic with the doctor, everything suddenly became a blur. He was unable to focus on what was being said, he heard the doctor's voice but didn't hear the words and he describes feeling frozen in time, being unable to make sense out of what he was being told.

Zena, who was in the middle of her admission assessment at the hospital, felt such an overwhelming sense of fear that she could not stay. She could no longer contain her fear and just wanted to go home to safety and, even though her husband said that he would not drive her home and that she had to stay, she retorted that she would walk, she would get a taxi, she was just going home, and home she went as fast as she could.

In conclusion then, the physiological response to crisis can be seen to affect people's thoughts, feelings, actions and reactions. These components of self are illustrated in the inner circle of the FRAGILE TEARS model of crisis as detailed in Chapter 1. Understanding how our biological self can influence how we respond to the world can enable us to be more effective in helping people experiencing crisis.

Activity

The physiological changes that take place when we are under stress can fuel amazing levels of energy. Can you recount any details or stories of people who have used this energy to good effect?

There are many anecdotal stories of people performing the most amazing feats to keep themselves safe. For example, someone losing a limb in an accident and being able to pick up the limb and run for help, or fighting sharks and beating off crocodiles are all things we would not believe ourselves able to do. Such is the power of the physiological response. Helping people cope with the fight or flight reaction and the physiological consequences of prolonged stress are discussed in Chapters 4 and 5 but now we move on to a behavioural explanation of our responses to stress and crisis.

A BEHAVIOURAL PERSPECTIVE

Behaviourists focus on our behavioural responses and, in particular, on what happens before, what happens during and what happens after behaviour. This is sometimes called the ABC of behavioural explanation: A = Antecedent, that which goes before; B = Behaviour, that which you can observe a person doing; and C = Consequence and what happens to the person after exhibiting that behaviour. For many years psychology has tried to find patterns of behaviour that were easily predictable on the basis that altering either the antecedent or the consequences of behaviour can help people change and adapt their behaviour to good effect.

The early contributors to behavioural psychology were the physiologist Ivan Pavlov (1849–1936), who used classical conditioning, and Burrhus Skinner (1904–1990), who developed operant conditioning. Behavioural models see the psychological problems following crisis as a vicious cycle of triggers, responses and consequences. The triggers could be internal, generated by the person themselves, such as thoughts and memories, or external triggers such as places, insects or animals. Our responses are the behaviours we have that follow a trigger and these responses may be to avoid the situation or to escape from it. Consequences are the result of the behaviour – for example, the reduction of anxiety feelings that a person gets when they avoid the situation or insect.

Classical conditioning

Classical conditioning is most concerned with Pavlov and his wonderful salivating dogs. Pavlov presented food to the dogs at the same time as a making a sound. The dogs gradually associated the sound with food and eventually salivated when they heard the sound. This model shows how everyday sounds and smells can be turned into traumatic stimuli because they are associated with the traumatic event (Gibson, 2006). For example, Martin describes being unable to drink cranberry juice although it was a drink he enjoyed in the past. During his treatment for cancer he noticed that the intravenous drug that they give him in the hospital looked just like cranberry juice. The colour of cranberry juice had therefore become associated with an unpleasant event for Martin.

Operant conditioning

Skinner proposed that reward and punishment were important in strengthening and weakening behaviour. If we are rewarded when performing a particular behaviour, we are likely to repeat the behaviour and if we are punished we will avoid the behaviour. Also, if punishment is stopped when we perform the behaviour we are more likely to reproduce the behaviour, and this is relevant in avoidance behaviour. Behaviourists suggest that we learn to be fearful and we learn how to manage that fear. One of the common ways people manage their fear is by avoidance but avoiding the situation is not a good way of dealing with an anxiety-provoking situation. Behaviourists suggest avoidance is how anxieties and phobias develop. When you experience bad feelings such as anger, fear, sadness or pain in a particular environment, such as at the dentist or the supermarket, you may seek to avoid this environment in the future, or the next time you are in the same environment you feel feelings of anxiety so you escape from the environment to lessen the anxiety. If we leave the supermarket or dentist when we feel anxious, our anxiety will reduce and avoidance is being reinforced. However, if the situation is avoided the anxiety about the place will increase so each time we avoid we become a little more afraid.

Habituation

Habituation is learning not to react to a stimulus that is consistent or not unusual in the environment. Habituation was a very relevant concept when I was working with problem drinkers and their families. What seemed like a crisis to me when I visited the family was not a crisis to the drinker or the family because it was not new. When the event first occurred it was perceived as a crisis. However, it had then become familiar and the family had incorporated their new crisis into the pattern of life.

COGNITIVE BEHAVIOURAL THEORY

The basis of cognitive theory is that although mental processes and meaning are personal and individual, a person can learn to act as a 'personal scientist'. Someone with a psychological problem that is interfering with them having emotional well-being can learn to question how they interpret their experience. People's emotional reactions and behaviour in crisis are strongly influenced by their thoughts and beliefs about themselves and the crisis situation (Westbrook *et al.*, 2007). Beck (1976) suggested that three levels of cognition operated in the maintenance of psychological disorder: negative automatic thoughts (NATS), dysfunctional assumptions and core beliefs.

NATS

NATS are commonly described as negatively charged thoughts or images, which flash through the mind, leaving an alteration in feeling. The identification of NATS may lead to recognising styles or habits of 'shorthand' unhelpful thinking, known as cognitive bias. There may also be positive and neutral thoughts that occur in a crisis and there are examples of these in the case studies in Chapter 2.

These are some examples of cognitive bias that influence how we operate.

Catastrophising	Exaggerates things, makes a mountain out of a molehill. Predicting a disaster without good evidence.	Rose: Dealing with the legal stuff is too hard; I will get it wrong and we will lose everything.
Filtered thinking	The individual 'filters out' all the positive things that have happened to him/her and only uses the negative things as points of reference.	Rose: while Spike was in hospital she recalls difficulties with his care – constantly worrying and thinking 'can't rely on them getting it right'. The phone would ring and she would get a mental image of him lying in bed with no drip or monitors working.
Arbitrary inference	The crystal-ball gazer – is clairvoyant and knows what will happen before he/she has even tried it.	Kate: it is no use asking for help – everyone else has their own things to deal with.
Dichotomous	Thoughts are rigid, things are seen in terms of 'all or nothing, right and wrong'.	Martin had thoughts that because he had the bad luck having cancer in the first place this meant it was not going to be cured.
Labelling	Often puts 'labels' on him/herself and others: 'coper, non-coper, good, bad, sick, well'.	Rose and Kate both saw themselves as copers, having self-control and being the mum for all the family; they cared for others before themselves.

Angel or devil	Must be perfect at all times; if not, he/she is useless. Unrealistic expectations and high standards.	Zena: 'I can't do the things I should be able to do; I am not the woman Alex married and he is better off without me.'
Generalisation	'It always happens to me . . . I never get the breaks . . . Whenever . . . Every time . . .'.	Zena: reflecting on her problems being fitted for an artificial limb, 'It always goes wrong for me, other people seem to get on OK.'
Emotional reasoning	Heart ruling head.	Martin remembers a very bad day he had on holiday in a tourist trap where he felt he had been fleeced. He sometimes has thoughts that that must be where his cancer started.
Fixed rules	The shoulds and should nots – often has overwhelmingly high expectations of him/herself. 'I should always be in control . . . I should never lose my temper. '	Kate: 'I must be the mum the one who cares for others'.

(Adapted from Norman and Ryrie, 2005)

NATS have the power to change a feeling (for example, from anger to fear) and they also have the power to increase or fuel bad feelings.

Dysfunctional assumptions

Dysfunctional assumptions are described by Bennett-Levy *et al.* (2004) as 'providing the soil from which NATS sprout'. They contain rules for living (or survival) with biased and often self-defeating specifications. Ellis (1994) described a similar concept, which he named irrational beliefs, the first two of which are the ones that I have found people most identify with.

1. I must be liked or accepted by every important person in my life, for almost everything I do.

The approval of others is pleasant but not essential. In order to live life fully we need to express ourselves, which means that at times we will do things of which others disapprove. If we are constantly trying to avoid disapproval we will either become passive individuals or people with a poor sense of self. If, despite our efforts, we are disapproved of, the result can be devastating, because our self-esteem is based on what others think of us (adapted from Ellis and Harper, 1975).

2. I must be successful, competent and achieving in everything I do if I am to consider myself worthwhile.

This means perpetually striving to do better and never being satisfied. Our value is directly equated to our achievements. The consequences are that we cannot relax, we feel useless if not working, and become perfectionists or immobilised by procrastination. We never achieve quite enough to feel really good about ourselves because there is always something else. Again the net result is dissatisfaction. It is important to overcome the fear of failure and to view failure as something actually helpful (Ellis and Harper, 1975). Bennett-Levy *et al.* (2004) suggests that both of these dysfunctional assumptions may be culturally reinforced.

Core beliefs

Core beliefs are usually learned early on in life as a result of childhood experiences (Bennett-Levy *et al.*, 2004). They are seen as the individual's 'bottom line', the deep structure underpinning our psychological being. Core beliefs are said to broadly fall into two types: 'I am unlovable' and/ or 'I am useless'. If the crisis event violates a core belief and cannot be handled by our positive beliefs then dysfunctional assumptions become more active, negative thoughts increase and result in unpleasant feelings; this is sometimes called a critical incident (Bennett-Levy *et al.*, 2004). Dattilio and Freeman (2000) give an example of Mary, who appears competent and achieving at work and has positive beliefs about her capabilities until she experiences a personal crisis situation and activates previously learned negative beliefs, which had been superseded by more positive beliefs. The negative beliefs such as 'I am alone' and 'I am incompetent' changed her behaviour and her work functioning suffered because she withdrew from people around her.

Figure 2 illustrates the two possible paths taken following a critical incident and the effect of negative and realistic thinking.

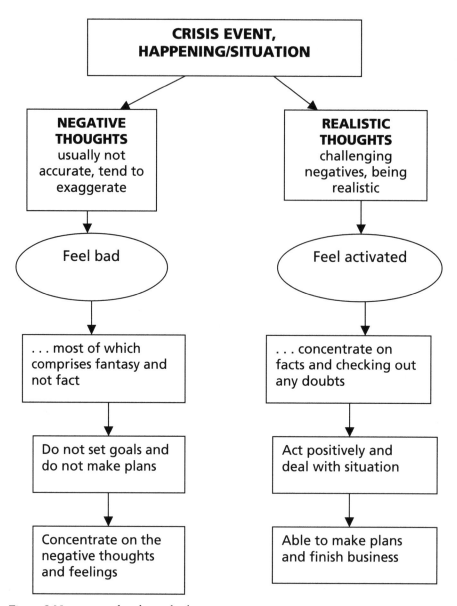

Figure 2 Negative and realistic thinking

Sometimes our perceptions of everyday events are skewed by our previous experiences. For example, Elizabeth recalls how she has overreacted to Tim developing a minor rash. Rather than thinking through the problem realistically – i.e., has he eaten something that has disagreed with him, is the rash a result of a change in washing powder, might it be a result of Tim using his new shower gel I bought for Christmas? – she automatically moves into negative thinking, exaggerating the situation by imagining that the rash is a sign of serious drug side-effects, that the drugs need to be stopped immediately and in doing so this will result in Tim having another seizure and that this time he might die.

The consequences of these negative thoughts are that Elizabeth then relives all the fearful feelings she had when Tim was seriously ill. The sense of helplessness and the overwhelming feeling of despair impact on her behaviour. However, she was able to recognise that the danger of staying with these thoughts and feelings is that she can become trapped into doing nothing and not taking any action to investigate Tim's situation further.

Elizabeth has learned to talk herself through these situations and, once calm, she is able to put her negative thoughts back in place and deal with the real situation, which is a young man who has a rash. Having challenged her negative thoughts, she takes charge of the situation. She books an appointment with the GP and makes sure she has all information at hand for the GP to assess the rash. The rash turns out to be short-lived and is gone in less than a week. This experience will help Elizabeth to be more rational next time something out of the ordinary presents itself and to see that her anxiety about Tim will fade as time moves on.

Elizabeth's experience is an example of how NATS can become a thinking habit, coming into the mind with no conscious effort, yet leaving a range of negative, mood-reducing feelings behind. NATS can also affect our mood as they take root and we ruminate over them. This continual replay of upsetting thoughts is like picking at a scab, painful yet compelling.

Activity

- Have you any experience of negative automatic thoughts?
- How did they affect your behaviour?
- How did they affect your feelings?
- What do you do to make sure that you appraise situations in a rational way?

PSYCHOANALYTIC THEORY

Psychoanalytical theory is the deepest of the theories for understanding mental distress because it is interested in the past. Childhood experiences are an essential component of who we are and have a great value in understanding feelings, especially unconscious feelings, and how they interfere with our present functioning. 'It is central to the psychoanalytic view that to be caught up in a severely traumatic event stirs up without fail unresolved pains and conflicts of childhood' (Garland, 2004, p. 4). Freud claimed that there are three levels of consciousness. An iceberg is often used to illustrate how much of the mind is unconscious, or under water, and so is not seen. Only a small percentage of the whole iceberg is visible above the surface (see Figure 3). The conscious mind is what we notice above the surface while the unconscious mind, the largest and most powerful part, remains unseen below the surface. At a conscious level we are aware of our thoughts and feelings. At our pre-conscious level we have memories and stored knowledge. The unconscious part takes up about 75 per cent of the mind and contains our fears, selfish desires, immoral sexual urges and violent motives. The unconscious part of our mind can be hinted at in slips of the tongue and in dreams.

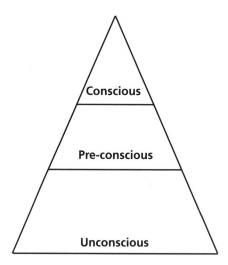

Figure 3 Three levels of consciousness

Sigmund Freud

Psychoanalysis was also the first of the theories that attempted to understand and explain mental distress. When we think of psychoanalysis we tend to think first of Sigmund Freud's theories. However, the psychoanalytic model has been evaluated, criticised and added to by other theorists including Jung, Adler and Klein. This section does not attempt to summarise all of the theories put forward by Freud and other psychoanalytical theorists, but to relate the theories contributing to understanding personal crisis.

Freud commenced his work in the 1890s by using hypnosis to treat neurotic patients. He was influenced by the work of Joseph Bruer. Freud suggested that there was a conflict between a memory and feeling that was trying to become conscious and another part of the mind that was refusing to accept the existence of the memory (Storr, 2001). Anxiety is an important concept in psychoanalysis; it is the warning system, the alarm bell that goes off when there are problems within the personality. Freud thought that a deep-rooted mental problem could cause current mental distress (Tyrer and Steinberg, 2005). Freud originally thought that the repressed memory and feeling began with an unpleasant or traumatic event that the person wanted to forget. To support this theory, more recent work with people who have post-traumatic stress disorder has shown that enabling a person to recover the memory and going through the event in detail helps the person recover (Storr, 2001). Freud later concentrated his work on sexual emotions which, if repressed, caused neurotic symptoms and he changed from concentrating on traumatic incidents to studying the sexual development of children. During the First World War Freud rethought his theory about anxiety based on war neurosis. Psychoanalysis became more recognised because of the treatment of war neurosis or shell shock.

The id, the ego and the superego

Freud suggested the personality comprised three parts and proposed his model of the id, the ego and the superego in 1923. This model helps to explain why memories and feelings are repressed.

The id	The id is seen as mostly unconscious. It is the part of us that is concerned with seeking pleasure and avoiding pain, it contains the libidinal and aggressive drives, it is the most primitive part, it is emotional, illogical and it is disorganised (Storr, 2001). Freud informs us that it contains everything that is inherited, that is with us at birth. Freud also states that we know little of it and the little we can access is through our dreams (Howard, 2006).	Your worst fears. Sometimes expressed in dreams or nightmares.
The ego	The ego is most concerned with self-preservation. It responds to external events by working out how to deal with them through memory, deciding whether to escape or to adapt and working out how to create a more positive environment. The ego acts as a go-between for the id and the superego. It responds to the internal conflict by gaining control over instincts (Storr, 1989; Bateman et al., 2000).	'Repress' your worst fears. Concerned with the practicalities and coping with the crisis.

| The superego | Gradually develops throughout childhood as a result of parenting; influence from parents and parent figures in society as a whole are gradually absorbed. The influences from parents and parent figures in the form of reactions to our behaviour and advice and criticism are gradually absorbed so that they become our own 'oughts' and 'shoulds' and we feel uncomfortable when we disobey them. | Judgemental voices in your head. 'It is all my fault.' 'If only . . .' |

Freud suggested that there were three causes for anxiety:

- the first is the real world, which includes traumatic events like crime, accidents, crisis and disasters;
- the second cause is the id – the instinctual feelings that demand fulfilment;
- the third is from the superego when we are fearful of being punished for a moral transgression.

Narcissism or self-love

In Freud's view the amount of psychic energy is limited and must be shared between all three parts of the personality. This explains why in a personal crisis too much energy is being used up trying to deal with unresolved conflicts. A healthy individual is able to resolve conflicts as they arise and therefore keep psychic energy for the ego to be able to develop and interact with the environment. The psychic energy associated with libido relates to a term Freud used, 'narcissism', which means self-love. It is a term that is often used in a negative way about a person and there is even a personality disorder named after it. However, a degree of self-love is very important to a healthy mind. Self-love could be said to relate to self-esteem, which is also very important for a healthy mind (Storr, 1989). Freud maintained that what matters in a healthy mind is the degree to which the libido is directed towards the self and the degree to which it is directed towards others. The libido is often associated with sexual drive. However, it can also be seen as a ball of energy or a motivational driving force. When you are 'in love' most of the libido is invested in the one that you love (Storr, 1989). When a relationship ends it could be said that you have to undergo a transition or crisis period when the libido moves from being invested in the other person to being invested in yourself or maybe another person.

Defence mechanisms

The table below lists some of the defence mechanisms described by Anna Freud and the psychoanalytical theorists that followed Freud. The table attempts to describe the defence mechanisms and to give real-life examples of how they are used to either keep away excessive anxiety or protect our self-esteem. The ego's ability to cope is what is needed in times of crisis; many of the ego defences could be seen as coping mechanisms.

Cramer (1998, p. 885) has adopted a working definition of defence mechanisms:

> The term 'Defence mechanisms' refers to a mental operation that occurs outside of awareness. The function of the defence mechanism is to protect the individual from experiencing excessive anxiety. According to older, classical psychoanalytical theory, such anxiety would occur if the individual became aware of unacceptable thoughts, impulses, or wishes. In contemporary thinking about defences, an additional function is seen to be the protection of self – of self esteem and, in more extreme cases, protection of the integration of self.

Anna Freud (1966) suggests that defence mechanisms are the way in which the ego wards off anxiety and upset and controls impulsive behaviour.

Defence mechanism	Description	Example
Projection	Parts of yourself that are split off and attributed to another person.	Husband displaces on to his wife his own impulses to be unfaithful and then accuses her of having an affair (Freud, 1966).
Denial	Not seeing the obvious; stating that it does not exist.	Ellie and her family denied Mae's continued illness.
Acting-out behaviour	Self-destructive, often repetitive behaviour.	Self-harming behaviour.
Hypochondriasis	The transformation of negative feelings towards others into negative feelings toward self, usually experienced as pain and illness.	Imagining that the symptoms of anxiety are in fact a major and serious health problem.

Regression	Going backwards to an earlier stage of development.	Having a temper tantrum when you do not get your own way.
Displacement	Expressing difficult feelings to a person or object that is less frightening.	Getting angry with your children when you are actually angry with your boss.
Intellectualisation and rationalisation	A person avoids uncomfortable emotions by focusing on facts and logic; making up a logical reason rather than facing the real reason why an event that is difficult to accept has happened.	On hearing that you have a serious illness, reading every source of information that you can find, or saying that the reason you were fired was because your boss did not like women when in fact it was due to your lateness and poor performance.
Repression	Placing uncomfortable thoughts and memories in areas of the subconscious mind.	Forgetting sexual abuse in your childhood.
Sublimation	Re-channelling of the psychic drive into constructive activity.	Creating works of art.
Suppression	The conscious decision to delay paying attention to an emotion or need in order to cope with the present reality.	Dealing with a crisis at the time and then, after the event, having an emotional reaction. Rose says that maybe it is the only way to deal with terrible news, 'not to let it in, keep active, manage the situation and then cry later'.
Humour	Laughing and joking when distressed.	This sometimes happens when firemen, police and others in emergency services deal with horrific events and make jokes about the circumstances.

People tend to have their own preferred defence mechanisms and these occur mostly involuntarily. Usually defence mechanisms are a healthy way of coping with anxiety but sometimes people in crisis, faced with overwhelming stress, will use defences in an unhealthy way.

TRANSACTIONAL ANALYSIS

Transactional analysis (TA) was created by Eric Berne and it became very popular in the 1960s. Berne wanted psychoanalysis to be accessible to everyone (Stewart and Joines, 1987). TA is still very influential in therapy, education and supervision. Transactional analysis theory, in my opinion, falls in between psychoanalytical theory and cognitive theory and incorporates many of the ideas of both theories. It explains a theory of how personality is structured in the ego state model, and the ego state model also helps us understand and analyse communication. TA offers a theory of child development with the explanation of a 'life script' – i.e. it shows us how our present life structure, beliefs and reactions originated in childhood.

The most relevant aspects of the theory to people in crisis are what TA describes as script development and the related themes of 'racket feelings' and 'drivers'. Transactional analysis describes the ways people interact when they communicate with each other and they do so from three ego states, which TA calls the parent, adult and child.

The parent ego state

The parent ego state is described by ITA (1999) as like a 'tape recorder – a collection of prejudged prejudiced, codes for living. When I am in parent ego state I hear a voice saying "stay strong, don't cry and try hard". The parent ego state is divided into nurturing parent and controlling parent (Stewart and Joines, 1987).

The adult ego state

The adult ego state is logical and able to solve problems. The child and parent feelings and judgements do not contaminate the process. The adult ego state is not divided.

The child ego state

In child ego state we act like we did when we were children. The child ego state is divided into free child and adapted child (Stewart and Joines, 1987). When we are in child ego state we are creative, spontaneous and also naughty; we are most likely to be in this ego state when we are at a party or a sporting event.

Throughout the day we can make many shifts from one ego state to another – Berne (1961) calls this a flow of cathexis. For a more detailed account of ego states and communication, read Donnelly and Neville (2008).

The existential position

Early on in life, around the age of three to seven, we start the process of deciding who we are. According to TA, at a very young age we make decisions about ourselves and others and these decisions are known as life positions. If we have a happy childhood and a good life we decide that we are OK. This is the healthiest and happiest position to be in and is called 'I am OK and you are OK'. However, we do not stay in the same life position throughout each day; we can shift position. When in a crisis situation it is possible that we move to one of the other less positive life positions. These include 'I am OK and you are not OK'; this is an angry position thinking that you are in the right and that someone else is to blame. Martin was briefly in this position when he got angry with his friends for smoking. 'I am not OK and you are OK' is a victim position and, lastly, the most negative position is 'I am not OK and you are not OK'.

Life script

A life script is a life plan and it is written by us when we are children. We write our life plan in response to what we see and experience in the environment and what we feel from the people around us, and also what is said to us directly or that we pick up indirectly from the important people in our lives. Our script is written in response to 'counter-injunctions', which are phrases that are actually said to us: for example, 'work hard', 'be good', 'do not tell lies' and 'be quiet'. Sometimes we will have the same messages from both parents but it is also possible to have direct commands from your father and conflicting commands from your mother. These direct commands come from our parents' parent ego state and it is very probable that they had the same commands from their parents.

Programme

We get 'programme' from our parents' adult ego state – this is where we pick up behavioural cues. We see children practising behaviours that they see in their parents; for example, a child telling her sister off in exactly the same tone of voice and using the same words that her mother does. It is likely that we pick up programme that relates to the counter-injunctions.

So, we are told to work hard and we see our father never taking time off work, going to work early and coming home late.

Injunctions and permissions

Injunctions and permissions come from our parents' child ego state. They are very seldom said but we experience them and they are implied by our parents or parent figures. Injunctions are negative and permissions are positive. Very often we will receive direct commands from our parents, we will see our parents performing the corresponding behaviours and we will feel the affects of pleasure and pain from our parents when we perform similar behaviours. Sometimes the script messages are confusing. For example, a father says to his son 'work hard', 'be clever', 'be successful', 'if a thing is worth doing it is worth doing well' and 'do not give up – try again'. These statements come from the father's parent ego state and are very likely to have been said by one or both of his parents when he was a child. The son saw his father work hard, he was aware that his father worked long hours and needed a drink of alcohol to unwind at the end of a long day. However, when the son passed his exams the father, although pleased, did not seem to celebrate the success. When the boy grows up the father listens impatiently to the boy's stories of achievement and immediately cuts in to tell a story of his own achievement. The counter-injunctions are clearly 'work hard' and 'be successful'; however, the child ego state in the parent is in competition and therefore the injunctions are 'do not be as successful as me'. In this situation there is the potential for crisis for the son as he becomes an adult.

The drama triangle

There are said to be three familiar roles played out in script behaviour. Karpman recognised these roles and devised the drama triangle. These roles are very evident in the crisis situations described earlier. The 'Victim' is not OK; they are discounted, bullied and abused. A victim is either persecuted or rescued. The 'Rescuer' helps the victim by doing something for them and the rescuer feels that they are OK and the victim is not OK. The rescuer discounts the victim's ability to rescue themselves. Kate describes the moment that she entered her parents' house: 'it was chaos, my daughter was crying, my mother was hysterical'. She states that she had to take charge for her child, for her mother and for her brothers. This role came naturally to Kate as she describes her childhood: 'I was the eldest; I had brought up my brothers from the age of eleven, my mum had severe depression and anxiety, she couldn't cope, she wasn't able to.'

People who work in the helping professions are often in nurturing parent ego state and therefore find the rescuer position in the drama triangle comes naturally. In many cases, when working with people in a crisis, it is appropriate to be in the rescuer role. However, we must be careful to recognise the person's ability to rescue themselves.

Lastly, the 'Persecutor' also believes the victim is not OK. The persecutor is the person who puts the victim down, bullies and abuses the victim.

During a crisis it is possible for people to switch positions on the drama triangle. For example, you start as a rescuer but exhaust yourself and become the victim. Another example is to try to rescue others who are also going through the crisis but this is viewed as bossy and unwelcome by others and you end up being viewed as a persecutor. Karpman describes a common example in a relationship: trying to help your partner with personal hints or unwanted advice that backfires quickly when he says 'now you, the rescuer, are the new victim'. Mitchell (2007) explains how two people alternated between the roles of victim, saviour (rescuer) and persecutor and describes her own experience as a victim of incest. She states that the victim has often been the abuser's emotional crutch (or rescuer) and she suggests that this pattern of relating often extends into adulthood, with the woman choosing abusive relationships where they are forced into the roles of victim, rescuer and sometimes even persecutor. For more examples of switching roles in the drama triangle, visit **www.karpmandramatriangle.com**

Racket feeling

Racket feeling is defined by ITA (1999) as a negative pattern of behaviour. I think of it as familiar bad feeling – a bad feeling that is felt in many different stressful situations. It has very little to do with the situation and it does nothing to solve my problem. A common example of a racket feeling is that of feeling we are stupid when someone asks you to solve a mathematical problem. Rather than think logically about the problem, we respond in a way that has more to do with our perception of ourselves and our negative feelings. We discount the adult ego state's ability to solve the problem and respond as an adapted child. We collect racket feelings like the Green Shield stamps that my mother collected in the 1970s or, nowadays, like club card points at the chemist or the supermarket. The racket system is how our life script is maintained. A racket feeling may also be a defence against a negative belief.

Drivers

TA theory suggests our behaviour, thoughts and feelings are driven by what are referred to as 'drivers'. We are most likely to see driver behaviour in others during a crisis. Drivers correspond with the counter-injunctions that have been mentioned earlier in script development. Kahler (1974, in Stewart and Joines, 1987) identified five drivers.

Key drivers	Self-assessment	Consequence
Be perfect People influenced by this driver will be purposeful, moral and have very high standards. They will be task-orientated and extremely logical.	Do you set yourself high standards and then criticise yourself for failing to meet them? Are you upset by small messes or discrepancies, such as a spot on a carpet and disorderly presentation of work?	As stress increases, the person will become more and more single-minded, seeing only their own point of view. They will become more and more controlling.
Please others People influenced by this driver love spending time with other people, and are comfortable in social situations. They are usually skilled in dealing with others, and like to look after people.	Is it important to you to be liked? Are you fairly easily persuaded? Do you dislike conflict? Would you normally avoid confrontation?	One of the most destructive aspects of this stress pattern is the urge to rescue anyone and everyone even if they do not need it.
Hurry up This person will be lively, adventurous, excited, often described as the 'life and soul of the party', enthusiastic, quick, with a capacity for doing lots of things at once.	Do you have a tendency to do a lot of things at the same time? Do you tend to talk at the same time as others, or finish their sentences for them? Do you like to 'get on with the job' rather than talk about it? Do you set unrealistically short time limits?	As the stress increases activity will become more and more frenetic.

Be strong		
People with this driver tend to be extremely stalwart in the face of difficulties and will carry on regardless.	Do you hide or control your feelings? Are you reluctant to ask for help? Do you have a tendency to put yourself (or find yourself) in the position of being depended upon?	Stress caused by: the fear of rejection through being seen as vulnerable; being 'forced' to say what they feel; exposing their weaknesses.
Try hard		
This person tends to take on lots of tasks. They set themselves high standards and are often viewed as hard workers.	Do you hate 'giving up' or 'giving in', always hoping that this time it will work? Do you have a tendency to start things and not to finish them? Do you tend to compare yourself (or your performance) with others or feel inferior or superior accordingly?	One of the main effects of stress is that much effort goes into trying but very little is achieved. Lots of tasks may be taken on, and promises may be made but something always seems to get in the way of a success.

(Adapted from Stewart and Joines, 1987.)

Activity

- What do you think that your driver behaviour is?
- Think about the case studies in Chapter 2. Which driver behaviours are being shown?

The most evident driver behaviour in the crisis stories in Chapter 2 is 'Be strong'. Kate shows this behaviour. Her self-talk at the moment of crisis was 'I had to take charge', 'I had to cope', 'I could not go to pieces'. She mentions that although she wanted her own space, she also wanted to help the rest of her family. She recalls feeling numb and cold and needing to squash the feeling of panic. Rose described going into overdrive; there was a lot to do so she had a burst of energy. Looking back at the time in hospital she worries that she came over to the health professionals as being too cold and unemotional.

GRIEF THEORY

Psychology attempts to understand and predict human behaviour and each of the theories discussed in this chapter uses a different approach to explaining thoughts and behaviour. That people respond differently to crises, stress and anxiety is now the perceived wisdom, but there are commonalities among people that, if understood in context, can be useful to us in dealing with or helping people cope with the emotional and psychological distress experienced in given situations. A good example of this is grief theory and the work of Elizabeth Kubler-Ross (1982) and the early work of Colin Murray Parkes (2006). They suggested that when people were exposed to a major life stressor, such as bereavement and loss, there were expected patterns of thoughts and stages of behaviour. In summary those stages/phases of behaviour included the following.

The shock and denial stage	The person may appear to be stunned by the news, not able to take in the information, being in shock. They may deny the information, refusing to accept it, accusing others of being wrong.
Anger and feeling stage	The person attributes blame to themselves and to other people, sometimes including the deceased and those who attempt to help. Emotions are high and crying is expected.
The acceptance stage.	The person realises that the situation is true and that their loved one really is gone, and starts to accept the loss as real.
Resolution	The person resolves their grief and moves on to building a future without them. The grief is resolved.

Activity

- Can you apply those stages of grief to any of the stories you have read in Chapter 2?
- Do the stages fit exactly or are there some inconsistencies?
- Why do you think that might be?

We now know that people do not follow such an orderly pattern of behaviour and that many people never really resolve their grief, they just become better at managing it, but many people exhibit some aspects of those behaviours described. We also know that some people appear to cope much better than others and that the ability of human beings to adapt to their circumstances has ensured their survival.

HUMANISTIC PERSPECTIVES

The humanistic approach suggests that when a crisis happens a person becomes aware of a lack of congruence within their concept of self and their experience. This means that our view of who we are has to change because of the experience of crisis. 'Congruence' refers to how things fit together within us – our thoughts and feelings correspond and agree with each other so there is a sense of balance and we feel we are in control. Rogers (1987) describes two mechanisms: distortion and denial. Distortion occurs when the individual perceives a threat to their self-concept so they distort the perception until it fits their self-concept. Denial follows the same process except that, instead of distorting, the person denies the threat exists. If we find ourselves in a traumatic situation our concept of self may become threatened and we will experience anxiety, such as the anxiety expressed by Ellie when she had to face the fact of Mae being deaf. Ellie moved from having a perfect child to having a child who will live her life as a deaf person. Elizabeth was in a similar situation: she had a perfect boy who was expected to live up to all her hopes and aspirations and now he was different and his surgery and the consequences of surgery will impact on the whole of his life experience. Zena also had to come to terms with a radical change in her appearance and physical ability. Although she fought hard to maintain her outward appearance and continued to engage in activities she enjoyed, she gradually realised she was unable to. The journey between realisation and acceptance is not straightforward and there are gains and losses along the way. All of these women had to face their fears, do battle with their attitudes and address previously-held values as they adjusted to the change in their lives.

The key theorist to mention here is Carl Rogers. He rejects the notion of labelling people and regards all people as unique individuals. Rogers (1987) said that experiences that are incongruent with self-structure are 'subceived' (perceived or anticipated) as threatening so the person will avoid accurate symbolisation of the threatening experience. For example, in Chapter 2 people in crisis stated, 'it's not real' and 'I'm in a bubble'. The person in crisis sees themselves as 'disintegrating', and may be confused, 'talking from different parts of the self'. For example,

Luke after his baby's death states 'part of me knows what is going on, part of me is scared and part of me wants to hide'. The person needs to make sense of life again, its symbols, personal meanings and integrate these into the new post-crisis life. Caplan (1964) argues that this is an individual working towards a state of emotional equilibrium; the concept of emotional homeostasis. A crisis will destabilise the equilibrium or the balance of self. We must either solve the problem or adjust to the non-solution.

As defined by Rogers, the conditions of worth are set up by our parents and other important figures in our life. We feel that we have to earn positive regard by behaving in a way that other people want. Conditions of worth are usually about the way we look, how well we do at school or at sport and how we behave to others. Conditions of worth force us to live according to other people's values rather than our own. Taylor (1983) defines crisis from the potentiality model, viewing the person in crisis as having self-curing ability as a major resource. For example, Alex repeating to himself 'It will get better, it's hard, but get on with it'. Opportunity for change is not about being 'positive', rather, it is the realisation that if the self-concept has been attacked, the conditions of worth and 'ideal' self may disintegrate under the pressure of inescapable reality – this is crisis. To recover fully from crisis we need to change. Effecting change is about our ability to build new conditions of worth and improve our self-concept. This is not an easy thing to do, which is why some people remain stuck following a crisis and for some professional counselling may be the only way forward. We provide another example of this in Chapter 4, where we explore Ellie's recovery through counselling.

Theories of crises can offer us no true answers and, like many theories, they are continuously being developed. Having a little knowledge of the theories that surround crises may help but, as a helper, you should never assume that you are always right. Common-sense psychology is the most you can aspire to offer unless you undertake extensive training and seek professional registration as a psychotherapist.

REFERENCES

Bateman, A., Brown, D. and Pedder, J. (2000) *Introduction to Psychotherapy: An Outline of Psychodynamic Principles and Practice*. East Sussex: Brunner Routledge

Beck, A. (1976) *Cognitive Therapy and Emotional Disorder*. London: Penguin

Bennett-Levy, J., Butler, G., Fennell, M., Hackmann, A., Mueller, M. and

Westbrook, D. (2004) *The Oxford Guide to Behavioural Experiments in Cognitive Therapy*. Oxford: Oxford University Press

Berne, E. (1961) *Transactional Analysis in Psychotherapy: The Classic Handbook to its Principles*. New York: Grove Press

Caplan, G. (1964) *Principles of Preventive Psychiatry*. New York: Basic Books

Cramer, P. (1998) 'Defensiveness and defence mechanisms'. *Journal of Personality*, December, 66 (6): 879–894

Dattilio, F.M. and Freeman, A.M. (2000) *Cognitive-Behavioral Strategies in Crisis Intervention*. London: Guilford Press

Donnelly, E. and Neville, L. (2008) *Communication and Interpersonal Skills*. Exeter: Reflect Press

Ellis, A. (1994) *Reason and emotion in psychotherapy*. New York: Birch Lane Press

Ellis, A. and Harper, R. (1975) *A New Guide to Rational Living* (rev. edn). Hollywood, CA: Wilshire

Freud, A. (1968)*The Ego and Mechanisms of Defence*. London: Hogarth Press

Garland, C. (2004) *Understanding Trauma: A Psychoanalytical Approach*. London: Karnac Books

Gibson, M. (2006) *Order from Chaos: Responding to Traumatic Events*. Bristol: Policy Press

Howard, S. (2006) *Psychodynamic Counselling in a Nutshell*. London: Sage Publications

Institute of Transactional Analysis (ITA) **www.ita.org.uk**

Karpman, S. **www.karpmandramatriangle.com** Accessed 28 March 2009

Kubler-Ross, E. (1982) *Living with Death and Dying*. London: Souvenir Press

Mitchell, R. (2007) 'Fix you?' *Therapy Today*, 18 (6): 12–14

Norman, R. and Ryrie, I. (2005) *The Art and Science of Mental Health Nursing*. Maidenhead: Open University Press

Parkes, C. M. (1996) *Bereavement: Studies of Grief in Adult Life*. London: Routledge

Rogers, C.R. (1987) *Client-centered Therapy: Its Current Practice, Implications and Theory*. London: Constable

Stewart, I. and Joines, V. (1987) *TA Today*. Nottingham: Lifespace Publishing

Storr, A. (1989) *Freud*. Oxford: Oxford University Press

Storr, A. (2001) *Freud: A Very Short Introduction*. Oxford: Oxford University Press

Taylor, S.E. (1983) 'Adjustment to threatening events, a theory of cognitive adaptation'. *American Psychologist*, 38: 1161–1173

Tyrer, P.J. and Steinberg, D. (2005) *Models for Mental Disorder*. Chichester: Wiley

Westbrook, D., Kennerley, H. and Kirk, J. (2007) *An Introduction to Cognitive Behaviour Therapy Skills and Applications*. London: Sage Publications

Chapter 4

Developing supportive interventions

This chapter introduces you to skills for caring for people in crisis including:

- applying theory to practice;

- the role of the helper;

- using a humanistic approach;

- psychodynamic interventions;

- cognitive behavioural approaches including CBT;

- the importance of self-awareness and reflection when trying to help;

- healthy living strategies;

- resources to support your learning.

APPLYING THEORY TO PRACTICE

The theories explored in Chapter 3 have provided explanations for the variety of behaviours we may see from people reacting to crisis. The lived experiences of the people we interviewed reinforce a core theme: a sense of being torn apart, the sense of self being shattered, a sense of being broken. In this chapter you will explore how theoretical perspectives can provide practical suggestions for ways in which we can engage with those in crisis.

We have all heard phrases such as 'being there for someone' and 'giving support' but what does this mean in reality? When you are with someone in crisis, how can you determine that what you are doing is helpful and what can you do if you have a strong emotional reaction, such as feeling lost, overwhelmed, frustrated or angry when you are supposed to be helping?

Crisis is not neat; it doesn't follow an exact pattern and it does not affect everyone in exactly the same way. We cannot offer an exact science or detailed approach to help you deal with crisis that will work with every person every time. But, there do appear to be certain key features that are present in many of us when faced with crisis and these are:

- dislocation;
- disbelief;
- fear of the future;
- self-doubt.

Those who told us their stories were able to identify helpful and unhelpful interventions. They recognised that the depth of emotion they experienced relating to the actions of others could change over time. For example, Rose recalls being 'furious' with medical and nursing staff when Spike went without analgesia and antibiotics for 24 hours while being transferred from an intensive care unit to a trauma ward. But later, she was able to identify with the staff concerned in the transfer and understood their difficulties. Kate recalls being initially irritated by people who wanted to tell her how they coped with their bereavement. However, with the passing of time she acknowledged that it can be reassuring to hear other people's stories, as it confirmed for her that she was normal in her reactions. Elizabeth described how she was exposed to the ordeals of others when in hospital with Tim, and how in the initial stages she believed nothing could be any worse than what she and Tim were experiencing and dismissed others around her. Over a very short period of time she realised that there were many with worse experiences than her own and she found comfort in knowing that Tim fared better than some.

Activity

- Can you identify experiences where others' responses to a person's crisis have not appeared particularly helpful at the time?
- What was the initial outcome?
- Did that change over a period of time?

Most of us can remember times when we have been given 'advice' or exposed to hearing other people's accounts of their own crisis that did not help at the time but perhaps, on reflection, did help later on, in that it helped to put things into perspective and confirm normality.

THE ROLE OF THE HELPER

So what is the role of the helper/practitioner at the time of crisis? There appear to be a number of roles that people can move in and out of, dependent upon the needs of the person in crisis. At different times we might be:

- Supportive;
- Anchor;
- Guide;
- Enabler

(SAGE).

Mearns and Cooper (2005) describe crisis as involving a response of 'dissonance', when the experience or perception of reality is affected by the crisis in such a way that the sense of self held by the person is under threat. The SAGE helper needs to use their interpersonal and assessment skills to recognise which SAGE element is most appropriate in their response. The people who told us their stories could clearly identify when other people used a helpful role. For example, Rose found her family supportive, Kate's husband was her anchor, Martin used the Macmillan nurse as his guide, and Zena was enabled to continue being active by getting a prosthetic limb which worked.

Being supportive

Being supportive involves providing things that give strength to the person in crisis. This support can be as simple as making a cup of tea and helping the person in crisis stay calm during a crucial period. It might involve providing a private space and tissues so that people can cry and it often involves ensuring that people are physically taken care of, including food, drink and rest. All Stella wanted in the early stages of her crisis was support and when people tried to give her more and made demands of her to tell her tale she withdrew.

Being an anchor

Being an anchor involves holding a person in place; making sure that the person is emotionally safe and comforted at times of stress. Partners are often best placed to act as an anchor in this situation. For Gill her father took the place of anchor when her husband was sent to prison and for Martin the love of his family held him firmly in place.

Being a guide

Being a guide operates on a cognitive level, providing information, helping people find the information that they need and advising them about what is available. As a helper you do not need to know all the answers, but having some insight into where to look for help can be of great value to the person in crisis.

Being an enabler

The role of enabler involves helping people regain a sense of control, to start to solve their own problems and helping them make things happen.

Maslow's hierarchy of needs (see Figure 1) demonstrates this quite well.

Maslow suggested that we all have needs that can be placed in a hierarchy and that it is the meeting of those needs that motivates our behaviour. In times of crisis we may not be able to meet those needs on our own and we may need help.

Activity

Using Maslow's hierarchy of needs, what kind of responses could you use to support a person in crisis?

Your response will reflect what you believe the person's needs to be. Perhaps you used the SAGE approach to identify the role you were playing. The key to effective helping is judgement, timing and interpersonal skills. More about that a little later.

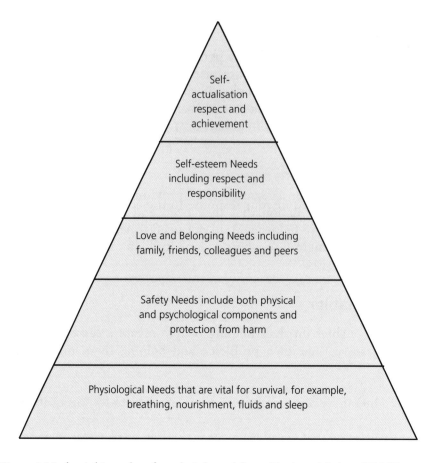

Figure 1 Maslow's hierarchy of needs (adapted from Abraham Maslow (1954))

USING A HUMANISTIC APPROACH

Some of you may see a person in crisis once only, while others will have continued contact with the person as they move through the experience. McLeod (2007) suggests even 10 minutes of contact can have an impact and he explains the idea of 'making a space', as a purposeful activity, to enable the person who is troubled or uncomfortable to use a 'counselling' space to reflect on other parts of their life, to regain perspective or gather inner resources for the next stage. Using the word 'counselling' here seems to imply that you are expected to enter into a formal therapy situation, but this is not the case.

Activity

- Can you recall a situation in which a person helped you through a period of distress?
- What did that person do to help?

Person-centred counselling

You may have included in your response to the activity things like: they listened, they gave me their time, they were kind, they seemed to want to help, they were non-judgemental, they put me first. All of these things are associated with helping and can also be considered to be skills of counselling. We can use a number of core counselling skills to build trust and establish rapport.

Activity

Can you identify and describe some of the core counselling skills?

You may have included:

- non-verbal communication, including facial expression, touch, posture, making sure your body and face are sending a message consistent with your words (congruence);
- respecting silence and how it contributes to building rapport;
- active listening, involving using open and closed questions, summarising and reflecting;
- basing your interactions on respect and genuineness, giving the other person your attention and acceptance;
- empathy and being non-judgemental.

It is likely that these terms are familiar to you, and that you are already skilled in some, if not all of them. Empathy and active listening are especially vital ingredients of communication during crisis. The effective helper can try to find out what is important to the person, his or her beliefs and perceptions about the situation and what they see as being the next step or immediate necessity.

Empathy

Person-centred counselling interventions explain the role of 'helper' as following the emotions and thoughts of the person in crisis, rather than attempting to direct or control them (Nelson-Jones, 2005). Empathy is a valuable quality and shows the person that they continue to be part of the world that is familiar, and that they are still worthy of being given time and the understanding of another person. A helper does not have to be an expert, but is someone who gives the other person a sense of being worthwhile and respected. Empathy has been described as the ability to imagine what it must be like to be in someone else's personal situation (Donnelly and Neville, 2008).

We might assume that someone in a helping role is able to be empathic, but this quality is not always in evidence. After going home from hospital, Zena needed practical help with daily living tasks. The only response from statutory services was an offer for someone to sit with Zena so her husband could go to the pub. Zena and Alex replied: 'We want to go together; we both enjoy the social aspect and pub quizzes. What is a stranger going to do sitting with another stranger for two hours? We need someone to help with the housework!' Rose was offended and angry when reading reports which said Spike was not as badly affected as was claimed: 'They never even saw him at home, never saw him confused or crying with pain.'

Active listening

Active listening involves accurate interpretation of meaning and a sensitive response to non-verbal communication, while taking account of the personal and social context of the exchange. Ellie described the experience of not being listened to; her fears were ignored, which added to the emotional confusion of Mae's illness and subsequent deafness. Bob recalls the realisation that he would go to prison: 'I felt like I was from another planet, not able to say what I felt, there weren't any words.'

The impression of distance is reinforced if there are no words to help us describe our feelings and thoughts. Active listening helps to bridge the gap between being 'frozen' and beginning to reach back into the world. Nelson-Jones (2005) has highlighted the vital role of active listening, 'Never being listened to is like a psychological death penalty'. Active listening involves summarising, reflecting back and paraphrasing. Using an internal frame of reference (that is: how you see, feel and experience the world) is a core active listening skill used for establishing a collaborative working relationship with the other person. Being able to respond from the other person's internal frame of reference (putting yourself in their shoes) can encourage them to explore the personal reality and implications of their own feelings, thoughts and actions.

Activity

Read the three situations given below and, in each case, identify which of the responses are from an internal frame of reference.

Zena 'My "friends" knew I was in hospital, then I let them know I was home, but they didn't call, visit or even send a card – that hurt.'

Responses:
1. 'Some people don't know what to say';
2. 'It sounds like you are better off without them';
3. 'You feel deeply hurt, you thought they cared, but they have not made contact'.

Martin 'They came round, then just started smoking, they knew I'd got cancer, I was so angry.'

Responses:
1. 'Didn't you tell them you were angry?'
2. 'You were angry and appalled at such insensitive behaviour';
3. 'You were angry, as you knew you had to take care of your health and they should too!'

Kate 'My mother can't cope since dad's death. I've tried to tell her how I feel, but she brushes me off'.

Responses:
1. 'Elderly people are like that, I'm sure she doesn't mean to get at you';
2. 'You feel frustrated because she doesn't seem to want to hear you';
3. 'You can't seem to get through, shall we role play this?'

Answers:
Zena: **Number 3**
Martin: **Number 2**
Kate: **Number 2**

Congruence

The helper is playing a part in supporting the person in crisis to move forward to a congruent sense of self. Being congruent involves being comfortable with who we are, with greater emotional and cognitive flexibility to be in touch with experiences (Donnelly and Neville, 2008). Greater acceptance of the sometimes oppositional or confusing 'parts' of the self begins the process of 'coming together', or mending.

Activity

What elements of the humanistic approach do you think that Kate, Martin and Elizabeth might have found useful?

These are some of our thoughts:

Kate – a friend just being with her when she cried, no words, just held her hand;
Martin – being able to be confused and ask 'silly' but important questions;
Elizabeth – having her deepest fears acknowledged.

Humanistic approaches suggest helpers are at their best when they show warmth, when they are truly genuine and use active listening skills, so letting the person in crisis have a safe space to vent feelings. The use of core person-centred interventions helps create a sense of safety and grounding for the person in crisis. This genuine demonstration of care has the potential to 'pave the way' for further contact.

PSYCHODYNAMIC INTERVENTIONS

Psychoanalytical theory may not seem at first to offer practical ways of helping individuals in crisis. However, Freud did offer an explanation for the development of dysfunctional behaviour and emotional distress. Howard (2006) reminds us that the unconscious is alive and it can kick. Psychoanalytical theory has evolved over the years and is now more commonly known as 'psychodynamic' to convey the idea of inner mental forces co-operating or, alternatively, at war. This has relevance for those in crisis, as actions and reactions to the crisis may be so unexpected as to cause them to fear 'losing it' and going out of control.

Control

The idea of control is viewed as a significant factor in psychological health (Walker, 2001). Control involves believing we are effective in what we do, and believing we can achieve what we set out to do. Walker also suggests that a balance of personal control and social support is desirable in time of crisis. For example, Zena's overall belief that she could regain more control of her life wavered at times. This was more noticeable when outcomes were dependent on things out of her control, such as getting a new false limb. Martin felt a lift in mood when he could take action, through exercise and improved diet, and Elizabeth felt much better when she knew she could take Tim back home.

Psychodynamic interventions usually take place over a long time period and may include the therapist being tuned into the client's unconscious clues, making interpretations to clarify the client's problem. Garland (2005) suggests 'the impact of a traumatic event upon the human mind can only be understood and treated through the process of achieving with the patient a deep knowledge of the meaning of that particular event for the individual'. You may remember reading about defence mechanisms in Chapter 3. Two important factors are active: firstly, that the defence mechanism may be used as a coping mechanism; and, secondly, it may have become a habit. The phrase 'If it ain't broke – don't fix it' comes to mind, in that we have already thought about ourselves and how we use defence mechanisms. We can decide not to do anything about a habit; but this decision may only be challenged if the habit outlives its use. Rose admitted she used 'being busy' as a way of putting aside feelings. She later wondered if this was as helpful as she had believed, as she may have given the impression she did not need any emotional support. During counselling Ellie became aware that she had been avoiding thinking about the impact of her daughter's deafness and this prevented her from fully dealing with her crisis. Ellie was using denial as a defence mechanism and was not able to move on until she had released the emotions and dealt with the practicalities of Mae's deafness. Through the counselling process Ellie was able to understand that her defence mechanisms were keeping her stuck; her counsellor encouraged her to explore her feelings and supported her when she expressed her feelings. Sometimes all counsellors have to do is to be there and listen, whereas at other times they may need to take on a more proactive approach. To find out more about counselling approaches we recommend that you visit **http://bacp. co.uk**, which is the website for the British Association of Counselling and Psychotherapy.

A psychodynamic therapist uses transference and counter-transference to clarify the client's inner world and the way in which the client experienced early relationships (Howard, 2006). Transference is where an individual transfers the thoughts and feelings that they have about another significant person in their lives onto the counsellor. For example, transference is the reason why some people respond to their counsellor as if they were their mother. Counter-transference is when the counsellor transfers those thoughts and feelings back to the person being counselled so, for example, the counsellor responds to their client as if they were their mother. This may be a deliberate or unintentional process. Transference and counter-transference of thoughts and feelings can be incredibly powerful and are extremely relevant concepts in the helping relationship during crisis. It is usually obvious to others that the person in the crisis is out of balance; they may appear and behave unlike their usual selves. However, the helper may also become out of balance, although recognising this may or may not come from within the helper. For example, during a panic attack in hospital Zena recalls a nurse saying briskly 'Don't be a silly girl, calm down.' Zena presented as a needy child and the nurse responded as an irritated mother as a result. Zena therefore had the feeling of being a child again, being ignored and denied choice. The nurse was not particularly helpful because she failed to see the consequences of her counter-transference. Had she been insightful she could have used the counter-transference to good effect, for example, by asking Zena to explore her thoughts and feelings at that time.

Activity

- When helping people through crisis what behaviours would you find difficult to deal with?
- Have you ever been unpleasantly treated or experienced a strong negative emotion when you have been trying to help?

Verbal and physical threat and aggression towards staff have become a constant concern in health and social care settings (National Audit Office, 2003). The person in crisis may have needs or be motivated by feelings which are not obvious to us or interfere with us doing our job. However, if that person's needs remain unsatisfied, this could create confusion, frustration or despair. We might not respond to these needs because we genuinely don't see or appreciate they are present. Also we may, on a conscious or unconscious level, decide not to respond because we don't believe we can cope. Coping includes the belief we have in our internal and external resources and motivation to engage with another person's distress. Emotion has healing properties. Psychodynamic approaches seek to 'open up' the levels of our conscious and unconscious feelings. This unblocking of emotional pressure offers an opportunity to get to know ourselves at a deeper level, moving towards greater self-acceptance.

In Chapter 2 we considered Monica's story. She, at the point of realising that her husband had been having an affair for some time, became extremely emotional; anger and despair were the predominant feelings. These emotions dissipated as she tumbled into despair. Monica's expression of emotions included damaging property, threatening to harm her husband and she expressed having violent dreams in which she stabbed the other woman and left her to bleed to death. Such emotion is difficult to manage in the helping situation as the intensity of emotion can frighten both the person and the helper. The key is for the helper to stay calm when the person is in this state and to facilitate a safe expression of emotions. Eventually the person will calm down, often as a result of exhaustion. Hitting pillows, shouting at empty chairs, tearing up newspapers, sobbing till it stops are all helpful ways to enable people to vent their feelings. When the process is near the end, they have expressed the emotion and are more able to see their crisis as a problem to be solved and not an emotion to be lived.

Using transactional analysis insights and interventions

Transactional analysis has developed as a more accessible psychodynamic approach and it offers insights and interventions that are easy to understand. The three ego states – parent, adult and child – clearly affect our responses to crisis. For example:

- in a parent ego state we could be nurturing, supportive and caring or critical;
- in an adult ego state we would be logical, capable and think rationally;
- in a child ego state we would be self-centred and highly emotional.

Activity

How might the telling of each story detailed in Chapter 2 be affected by each of the ego states?

We thought of these:

Parent: the person would recognise a need for support, accept help or care if offered and appreciate being treated with compassion.

Adult: the person would sort out what happened into accurate timelines, recognise their own role in the events, reflect on decisions and attempt to view events with balance.

Child: the person would express strong emotions, hurt, loss, fear, sadness, anger.

Activity

- How do our lists compare?
- Now consider how you could support or enable a person in crisis to express themselves in each of the ego states.

Driver behaviour

In Chapter 3 we introduced the concept of 'driver behaviour' and suggested that people in crisis are most likely to resort to their habitual driver behaviour. As a crisis worker we need to understand that the person in crisis is following deep-rooted and well-rehearsed patterns of behaviour. The following table illustrates some strategies for helping and responding to a person in the initial stages of crisis. An 'allower' is a positive balancing statement that you can say to a person or encourage them to use when they are in the grip of driver behaviour.

Driver	Helping to reduce stress in others	Allower	Example
Be perfect This person wants what they have done to be valued.	Always keep appointments and turn up on time. Reassure the person that they are not at fault, do not play down their concerns, acknowledge and praise their achievements.	You are good enough as you are.	Rose: when reporting on her husband's physical state to medical staff she gives a full report, worried that she will miss important details and, as a nurse, she should get it right.

Please others This person wants to be valued for who they are.	Express genuine regard for them as a person, keep your cool and remain polite even if you feel angry with the person. Unless you are able to enter into a deeper level of interaction, keep it simple.	Please yourself.	Kate: believing that she should always look after her family's emotional and material needs before her own.
Be strong This person does not want to appear vulnerable.	Do not take them for granted. Do not pressure them to express emotion. Be direct about what you would like to happen, avoiding emotionally laden language and double meaning.	Be open and express your wants.	Alex: waiting around in hospital was difficult because he had no role. He was eager to do jobs such as get coffee and buy nightclothes.
Try hard This person wants to be seen as doing the right thing.	Praise the person for finishing tasks, be constructive yet firm in supporting them in completion of tasks. Avoid conversation around comparison with others.	Do it.	Bob continuously made lists of his outgoings, put them away and did nothing to address the core problem.
Hurry up This person wants to be seen as busy.	Acknowledge the person's competence, try not to be put off by their way of letting off steam. Let them know you appreciate them slowing down.	Take your time.	Elizabeth: she was hypervigilant and ready with criticism when she perceived poor or just good enough care.

(Adapted from Stewart and Joines, 1987)

COGNITIVE BEHAVIOURAL APPROACHES

Self-doubt, fear of the future and doubts about ability to cope were all highlighted at the start of this chapter, and remained as key themes for the people we interviewed. We do not have magic wands to make everything OK again, the 'if only' wish is a very human trait. The SAGE helper aims to offer support and 'anchoring', but may also recognise a time to be more directive in their interventions. The 'guide' and 'enabler' roles call for tentative and gentle questioning skills, with the aim of opening up the person in crisis to considering changes in daily routines or styles of thinking. Cognitive behavioural therapy (CBT) can contribute to a person's efforts to regain some control over what can seem chaotic.

Thoughts and feelings interact, with the resulting behaviour being helpful or unhelpful. Separating thought, feeling and behaviour may seem artificial, as these are all aspects of what make up 'me' and are intertwined (Westbrook *et al.*, 2007). However, CBT aims to discover how a person's difficulty works, and how it is maintained. The person in crisis has to survive, for themselves and/or because they have others to support, materially and emotionally. The helper may need to engage with the person as guide or enabler. Making decisions, making choices, taking action may all seem immense hurdles while in deep distress. A guide can give information, such as where to go for specific help, or help with working through the decisions and consequences. Two aspects in particular can aid the process: flexible thinking and self-soothing.

Self-soothing techniques

These are easy and include things that make us feel better. Thinking nice thoughts, recalling happy memories, counting your blessings, taking a walk in a pleasant environment are all ways of soothing jangled nerves and tense bodies. Relaxation techniques discussed later in the chapter are an effective way for calming and relaxing the body and the mind.

Flexible thinking

Avoiding 'shoulds' or 'oughts'

Flexible thinking includes avoiding 'shoulds' or 'oughts' and other rules you may follow, without revising them, especially in light of changes in circumstances. In the enabler role, a helper can ask gentle, open questions. For example, Kate felt she 'should' look after her children, her mother and her brothers' emotional needs. She also felt the need to care by insisting the family had cooked meals every night. Her husband asked 'Would we love you less if we had a take-away together once a week?' She then began to realise she could let go of some of the tasks she gave herself. Rose had many phone calls, cards and letters from friends and colleagues, which was, for her, 'some light in the grey'. She began to feel guilty that she had not had time or energy to reply to them all. Her daughter asked, 'It would be nice to reply to them all, but do you believe anyone will think less of you if you don't?'

Self-acceptance

Neenan and Dryden (2002) point out that, without being accepting of oneself as a fallible human being, there are risks that we leave ourselves open to psychological self-harm. This happens when we give ourselves 'put-downs' or negative messages, for example, 'I'm no good at putting over my views', 'I'm too thick to understand this'. Zena had visits for assessment for daily living aids. At first she found dealing with professional health and social care personnel daunting. However, she realised that if she did not explain her needs and give her opinions, she would not get the most useful aid and public money would be wasted. She said, 'I know me and what makes me tick, and I'm happy with that – if other people aren't, that's not my problem.' Ellie avoided asking too many questions when Mae was first ill, as she thought the health care professionals must know more than she did: 'I'm just a new mum.' She later felt very guilty that she could possibly have let Mae suffer for longer than necessary through believing herself lacking in experience as a mother.

Activity

Review the reading in Chapter 3 on cognitive bias – our thoughts, assumptions and beliefs (see page 61). Can you think of three examples and the ways in which they could affect how someone copes during crisis?

You may have included the following cognitive biases.

1. Arbitrary inference – 'crystal ball gazing', knowing what will happen before you try it. This could be unhelpful because this thinking bias prevents trying something different, such as asking for help or changing a habit. It could also feed the belief that life is hopeless, as nothing can ever be changed.

2. Catastrophising – the worst will happen, you make mountains out of molehills. This could stop someone making any effort at all; helplessness sets in, or stokes anxiety beyond a level needed for energising into action.

3. Fixed rules – the 'shoulds' and 'oughts' – reflect high expectations of self and others. These rules reduce coping ability as they put added pressure on the self to 'get it right', or can increase frustration or disappointment if others don't behave as you believe they 'ought'.

CBT is broadly based on the idea that what you think about events and situations in your life affects your feelings (Neenan and Dryden, 2002). This is relevant for those in crisis as their usual balance is disrupted, and unhelpful thinking that is already established can be made worse by increased fear and sadness. The initial shock and necessity for dealing with practical issues may be followed by a time of facing consequences. Relationships may have to be renegotiated, the self-concept reviewed, values and beliefs re-evaluated. Those directly involved in the crisis may also have to deal with how others significant to them have reacted to the crisis and to changes in the pattern of life. Zena was hurt and angry that some friends ignored her; Stella had mixed feelings of relief and rejection; Kate realised there was a deep hole in her life and yearned for her father; Luke found joy and satisfaction in appreciating the love and support of his family.

THE ROLE OF SELF-AWARENESS AND REFLECTION

Reflection is vital as part of our learning and continued confidence in ourselves as care givers. Being skilled in the use of competent, compassionate and constructive helping skills will, if we are open and honest, bring us closer to those we encounter. I am sure you have gathered from the narratives of those we interviewed that the humanity of those they deal with made a significant difference in many ways. Yet, witnessing another person being in distress and anguish takes its toll, as does being in distress yourself. Being alert to our own stress 'early warning signs' is not a luxury or an optional extra. Kate recalls becoming seriously ill because she denied what her body was telling her. Alex ended up having surgery because he pushed himself to the limit of his physical capability.

Reflection

Becoming more aware of signs of stress involves reviewing our thinking, physical and emotional feelings, and behaviour. What are you aware of in these four areas that indicate you might be going 'overdrawn at the energy bank'?

You may have noticed:

Thinking: not able to concentrate, difficulty in making decisions.

Physical feelings: tired all the time, flatulence, aches and pains.

Emotional feelings: easily irritated, lack of enthusiasm, moody.

Behaviour: 'can't be bothered', less sociable.

Wilson (2006) notes that burnout is a real risk, especially if early warning signs are ignored or denied. If you become overly stressed, you may reduce your ability to help others. This does not imply you don't care, can't be bothered or have more important things to do – it does suggest you are human. Look again at some of the things people used to help during their experience of crises, and then look at the next section of this chapter. One aspect of the helpful strategies was taking time for oneself, just to read or take a fragrant bath or go for a walk. We all need time to process events, emotions and thoughts; even water takes time to digest. Making a little space to do this allows us time to re-evaluate and refresh ourselves.

Self-development opportunities

You might want to consider further self-development as a helper by committing yourself to a counselling course, engaging with therapy, or attending workshops that focus on specific aspects of self, such as assertion or creativity. Your organisation might offer supervision, on an individual basis, or as peer or group supervision. There are a number of ways of delivering supervision, all of which should offer support and development.

HEALTHY LIVING STRATEGIES

In order to avoid adding to problems during a crisis it is important to eat a healthy diet, get enough sleep and do some sort of physical activity regularly. These are the basics to keep your body functioning at its best. The way in which we live, what we eat, how much we sleep, rest and exercise has a significant effect on how we feel and how much we can do. 'A healthy mind in a healthy body' is an old chestnut but worth taking on board. Being healthy contributes towards feeling content and able to react constructively to adversity. If you cannot achieve a healthy balance in your lifestyle and you have, for example, a poor or unbalanced diet, insufficient physical activity, overuse of alcohol, illicit drug use, excessive worry, keeping strong emotions locked inside – you are more likely to have difficulty concentrating, making decisions, dealing with life's annoyances and recognising when you are heading towards more serious physical or psychological difficulties.

Activity

How healthy is your lifestyle? Take a moment to reflect on the past few weeks.
- What is your eating pattern?
- How much water do you drink in a typical day?
- How much alcohol do you drink a week?
- How much exercise do you engage in?

Nutrition

The Mental Health Foundation and Sustain have joined forces to launch the Food and Mental Health Campaign. The aim is to explain to people that the foods they eat can affect their brain and therefore their mental health (**www.mhf.org.uk/campaigns/food-and-mental-health**). The brain is sensitive to what we eat and drink and food affects how we feel, think and behave. Most of us are aware that smoking, drinking alcohol and tea and coffee can have a temporary mood-changing effect. However, Geary (2001) believes 'greater understanding of your moods and energy levels is possible through exploring the links between diet, nutrition and emotional and mental health'. Geary (2001) has worked with people of different ages on changing their diets and they noticed improvements in their mental health including lower levels of anxiety and depression, fewer cravings and less fatigue.

Food type	Found in	Effect on mood
Caffeine	Tea, coffee, chocolate, fizzy drinks.	Helps us stay alert and keeps us awake. Causes irritability and poor concentration.
Whole grains	Beans, fruit, vegetables, nuts, seeds.	Can help to keep cravings under control.
Oil-rich fish	Mackerel, herring, pilchards, sardines, salmon and fresh tuna.	Tryptophan can be converted into the mood-enhancing brain chemical serotonin. Hibbeln (1998) noted that countries with high fish consumption had lower levels of depression.

Sugar	Table sugar added to tea, coffee and breakfast cereal. Natural sugar from fruit and vegetables.	Brain cells use five times more sugar than other cells, so are very sensitive to changes to blood sugar level. Refined sugars can create a 'roller coaster' ride.
Water	From the tap or bottled.	Our body is about 3/4 water and we need about 8 glasses of water a day to replace what we lose and avoid headaches from the effects of dehydration.
Fat	Omega 3 essential fats from fish, oils such as linseed oil, walnuts.	The brain is 60% fat so it is important not to cut fat out of your diet. Low-fat diets can contribute to anxiety and depression.

Geary (2001) suggests an excess of meat, eggs, cheese and salt can create a craving for foods such as alcohol, juices, coffee and sugar to regain a balance. The government suggest that three or more units of alcohol a day is unhealthy for women and four or more units a day is too much for men. The recommended weekly drinking limits of 21 units of alcohol for men and 14 for women was first introduced in 1987. A unit is equal to half a pint of beer, a single shot of spirits and a small glass of wine.

Brain chemicals influence the way we behave and they can be affected by what we eat, and sugar is an example of a food that affects brain chemistry. Not all sugars are bad; natural sugars from fruit and vegetables do not create the highs and lows that the sugars from sweets can produce. Eating breakfast in the morning is recommended to establish an even blood sugar throughout the day.

Physical activity

The benefits of physical activity have been well researched in several different mental health and physical problems. Faulkner and Taylor (2005) present and discuss the psychological benefits of activity in several health-related areas including schizophrenia, drug and alcohol rehabilitation, cancer, smoking cessation and sleep. Martin reported how he felt after being diagnosed with cancer and while waiting for his first treatment, 'All of this time I am feeling fine, I am not unwell, it was three weeks until I had the first treatment. They said, "build yourself up and get strong", I took that to heart. That was something that I could do to deal with it, I felt really good.' The specific quality-of-life benefits of being active while being treated and after treatment for cancer are many. Courneya (2003) reported on nine studies that examined the benefits of exercise for people being treated for cancer; people who engaged in an exercise programme were compared with a control group who did not participate in exercise. Improvements included reduced pain, increased vigour, reduced fatigue, less nausea, and general increase in well-being and satisfaction with life.

Martin seems to have set great store by this advice: 'I keep a record of how many times I go for a walk. I went out for a couple of hours but I was worried that I had done too much.' In large population reviews people report that exercise promotes sleep and reliable effects were noted by people doing one hour of exercise a day. The type or intensity of exercise did not seem to matter. Disturbed sleep is a common problem with people who are in crisis and insomnia can bring about more problems, especially with the use of prescribed or non-prescribed medication to help get some sleep. Alcohol may seem a solution, especially as it is socially acceptable and easily available. Sleeping pills are associated with dependency and many side-effects such as nausea and daytime sedation (Kripke, 2000). One of the ways in which physical activity may promote sleep is by its anti-anxiety and antidepressant effects. O'Connor *et al.* (2000) suggest the evening may be the best time for exercise as the main anti-anxiety benefits are in the first few hours after doing physical activity.

Relaxation

There are sound reasons for learning how to use relaxation during crisis. When we are in a crisis situation we are likely to be in a state of high anxiety. During a crisis we need to be thinking clearly, making important decisions and concentrating on and dealing with the facts, which are very difficult things to do when we are feeling extremely anxious. In Chapter 3 we explored the physiological effects of anxiety and the concept of fight, flight and freeze. In a flight-or-fight situation our breathing becomes shallower and fast, our thinking may be negative and irrational and our feelings and behaviour are also detrimentally affected. We have control of our breathing, our thinking and our behaviour and, by controlling one of these areas, we can affect change in other areas and ultimately change how we feel and therefore how we deal with the situation. Relaxation produces changes to our body that are the opposite of the fight-or-flight reaction. Relaxation reduces sympathetic and increases parasympathetic nervous system activity. Relaxation lowers the heart rate, reduces blood pressure and sweat gland activity. It is important to note that when we are in a high state of anxiety it is difficult for us to let go of our tension; it feels like a mental and physical battleground. Our body does not want to release the tension, almost as if we feel more vulnerable without the tension. Therefore, when we most need it we have to convince ourselves to use the techniques and persevere with them. Relaxation is a skill that needs to be learned and practised.

Overview of relaxation techniques

There are many types of relaxation, some lasting a few minutes and some lasting an hour. Relaxation techniques can be done sitting in the chair or in the car stopped at a red traffic light, and it can be done standing up or lying down. It is easier to achieve full relaxation when you are lying down and comfortable with no interruptions. However, when you are in a crisis situation you do not often have the time and the shorter relaxation techniques are still useful.

Breathing exercises

Herbert Benson's (1975) relaxation response meditation technique is concerned with controlling breathing. It is quick and effective: 'The relaxation response is a physical state of deep rest that changes the physical and emotional responses to stress... and the opposite of the fight or flight response' – see **www.relaxationresponse.org**

Deep muscle relaxation

Progressive muscle relaxation (PMR) is a widely used relaxation method that was originally developed by Jacobson in 1938. In this technique, you focus on slowly tensing and then relaxing each muscle group. This helps you focus on the difference between muscle tension and relaxation, and you become more aware of physical sensations. You may choose to start by tensing and relaxing the muscles in your toes and progressively working your way up to your neck and head. Tense your muscles for at least five seconds and then relax for 30 seconds, and repeat.

Autogenic relaxation

Autogenic therapy, or AT, was developed in the early years of the twentieth century by the psychiatrist and neurologist Dr Johannes Schultz. 'Autogenic' means something that comes from within you. In this technique, you use both visual imagery and body awareness to reduce stress. You repeat words or suggestions in your mind to help you relax and reduce muscle tension. You may imagine a peaceful place and then focus on controlled, relaxing breathing, slowing your heart rate, or different physical sensations, such as relaxing each arm or leg one by one (see: **www.autogenic-therapy.org.uk**). The relaxation method can follow the same procedure as the progressive muscular relaxation and, instead of tensing the muscles, you concentrate on the muscle groups.

Guided fantasy relaxation

A guided fantasy relaxation is a mental journey to a beautiful place taken while being guided by a soothing voice on a tape or CD. You are asked to imagine a natural scene – a garden, a meadow or a beach. In a garden you may be directed around a path and asked to look at the plants and flowers and appreciate the variety of colours, you may be encouraged to smell the freshly cut grass and feel the warm air on your skin (Payne, 1998).

Meditation

There are many schools of meditation. One concept that links them is the process of emptying the mind of thoughts. You focus your attention on an object, sound or other experience such as a breath, candle, part of the body or a word (Payne, 1998).

One strong and constant theme from the narratives of 'our' people in crisis and from theoretical perspectives has been that of confidence. This is confidence in the competence of the person giving help, but also the confidence of the helper in their own competence and emotional ability.

The hope of those who have fought through a crisis is for 'calm waters', reaching a state of being which acknowledges the radical changes forced on them by their experiences. However, despite the passage of time and putting a great deal of effort into making meaningful change, balance may elude some individuals. The distress may continue and become entrenched, reducing ability or desire to engage in everyday life. In the next chapter, we will find out more about longer-term reactions to crisis, such as depression, anxiety or post-traumatic stress disorder.

RESOURCES

Further information about CBT is available on the following websites:

www.babcp.com

www.psychnet-uk.com/psychotherapy/psychotherapy_cognitive_behavioural_therapy.htm

If you want to get a deeper appreciation of CBT, or wonder if your thinking habits might be unhelpful, look at the self-help websites:

www.feelgood.com

www.themindgym.com

www.livinglifetothefull.com

The 'Overcoming' series of self help books, based on CBT techniques, includes titles covering, for example: depression, low self-esteem, eating disorders, phobia and anger management –
see **www.constablerobinson.com**

Relaxation website –
see **www.ptsd.org.uk/relaxation.htm**

Nutrition website –
see **www.mhf.org.uk/campaigns/food-and-mental-health**

The National Debt Line has a great deal of practical help and information available online or over the phone –
see **www.nationaldebtline.com**

And the BBC has information regarding financial issues –
see: **www.bbc.news.org**

Professional code of conduct
British Association for Counselling and Psychotherapy: BACP (2007)
Ethics for Counselling and Psychotherapy –
see: **www.bacp.co.uk/ethical-framework**

REFERENCES

Benson, H. (1975) **www.relationresponse.org**

Courneya, K.S. (2003) 'Exercise in cancer survivors: An overview of research'. *Medicine and Science in Sports and Exercise*, 35 (11): 1846–1852

Donnelly, E. and Neville, L. (2008) *Communication and Interpersonal Skills*. Exeter: Reflect Press

Faulkner, G.E.J. and Taylor, A.H. (2005) *Exercise, Health and Mental Health*. London: Routledge

Garland, C. (2005) *Understanding Trauma: A Psychoanalytical Approach*. London: Karnac Books

Geary, A. (2001) *The Food and Mood Handbook*. London: Harper Collins

Hibbeln, J.R. (1988) 'Fish consumption and major depression'. *Lancet* 351 (9110) 1213.102

Howard, S. (2006) *Psychodynamic Counselling in a Nutshell*. London: Sage

Jacobson, E. (1938) *Progressive Relaxation*. Chicago: University of Chicago Press

Kripke, D.F. (2000) 'Chronic hypnotic use: Deadly risks, doubtful benefit'. *Sleep Medicine Reviews*, 4: 5–20

Maslow, A.H. (1954) *Motivation and Personality*. New York: Harper and Row

McLeod, J. (2007) *Counselling Skill*. Maidenhead: Open University Press

Mearns, D. and Cooper, M. (2005) *Working at Relational Depth in Counselling and Psychotherapy*. London: Sage

National Audit Office (2003) *A Safer Place to Work: Protecting NHS Hospital and Ambulance Staff from Violence and Aggression*. London: Wiley

Neenan, M. and Dryden, W. (2002) *Life Coaching: A Cognitive Behavioural Approach*. Hove: Brunner-Routledge

Nelson-Jones, R. (2005) *Introduction to Counselling Skills* (2nd edn). London: Sage

O'Connor, P.J., Raglin, J.S. and Martinsen, E.W. 'Physical activity, anxiety and anxiety disorders'. *International Journal of Sport Psychology*, 31, 136–55

Payne, R.A. (1998) *Relaxation Techniques: A Practical Handbook for the Health Care Professional*. London: Churchill Livingstone

Stewart, I. and Joines, V. (1987) *TA Today, A New Introduction to Transactional Analysis*. Nottingham: Lifespace Publishing

Walker, J. (2001) *Control and the Psychology of Health*. Buckingham: Open University Press

Westbrook, D., Kennerley, H. and Kirk, J. (2007) *An Introduction to Cognitive Behaviour Therapy: Skills and Application*. London: Sage

Wilson, E. (2006) *Stress Proof Your Life*. Oxford: Index Books

Chapter 5

Crash or change

Key themes

This chapter introduces you to:

- outcomes of crisis;

- change and transition;

- blocks to resolution;

- working within a legislative and ethical framework;

- mental illness;

- post-traumatic stress disorder (PTSD).

OUTCOMES OF CRISIS

In Chapter 1 we introduced the FRAGILE TEARS model of crisis, which included three illustrations: pre-crisis, crisis and post-crisis. To aid our discussion about the outcomes of crisis we will be using the post-crisis illustration (see Figure 1).

Crisis impacts on a person's thoughts, emotions, actions and reactions. The self, when under threat, is often in disarray and the outcome of experiencing a crisis is that the person is changed. Figure 1 depicts that change as dislocated joints within the inner circle properties. The disjointed sections are mended but scars remain. We offer the following analogy to aid understanding: fractured bones heal, damaged skin knits back together and a broken pot can be mended but they are all left with 'scars' where they are joined. The 'scars' can become really tough or they may be an area susceptible to further damage. People are self-regulating and the joints in the diagram represent the 'scars' left by crisis. Following crisis some people become incredibly resilient as they 'toughen up', or

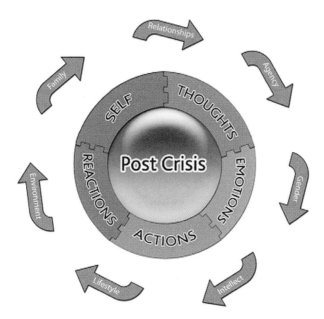

Figure 1 FRAGILE TEARS model post-crisis

they may become vulnerable to further damage. A good example of this is Gina, whose home has been flooded on three separate occasions. On the third occasion she knew exactly what to do to protect her belongings and she responded in a very proactive way to limit the damage to her home and save her precious items. Gina's mother, who lives in the same area, has found each flooding worse than the last and she has become increasingly distressed, which has impacted on her overall health. Gina and her mum are now protected by newly built flood defences but the experience of crisis has changed them and their outlook on life.

Many of the people we worked with, when reflecting upon their crisis, recognised that if the crisis had never happened many other positive events would not have taken place. They all agreed that they had changed in some way, with some thinking themselves to be stronger than they were before the crisis while others intimated that they had become more vulnerable as a consequence of the crisis experienced. The personal crisis experienced by those who shared their stories with us was said to be a 'powerful' event during which they were out of control. Surviving and existing after crisis involves change and taking back control, not least because beliefs, rules and assumptions which directed their lives are reviewed and questioned.

CHANGE AND TRANSITION

Change can involve a major shift in habits such as leaving a long-standing relationship, or a seemingly minor change such as remembering to take recycled bags back to the supermarket.

Activity

- Have you ever tried to change something significant in your life?
- What prompted you to make the change?
- Was the process of changing something easy or difficult for you, and why?

Some themes you may have noticed when considering your change may include outside influences. For example, changing a health-related aspect of behaviour may be in response to the latest health promotion campaign or may be because you want to make an impression on another person. Whether the experience of making a change to your life was easy or difficult is dependent upon many variables. Motivation, personality, support mechanisms, rewards and having people in place to help when the going gets tough all help in the process of change. Having a clear idea of what you want to achieve enables you to put things in place to action your ideas and it feels good when you get where you wanted to be, but instigating change when you are experiencing a powerful event in which you are not in control is a daunting task.

The saying 'old habits die hard' is especially meaningful during crisis. Old habits may include routines, such as going to work, or 'fun' things like the cinema or gardening. The outer FRAGILE ring of the crisis model contains more variables we have to address during those changes. The outer FRAGILE ring contains many potential impersonal factors that can all impact on how we respond to crisis. During the initial phases of crisis, there is usually an allowance made for the power of emotional reaction over the more rational course of planned action. We would not normally expect a person in crisis to act in a rational, consistent way. There are big variations in the use of coping skills and our ability to contain emotions and use levels of constructive problem-solving. Breaking down a problem or difficulty into bite-sized pieces can help to make the difficulties encountered in change and transition less daunting. Hopson *et al.* (1988) suggest there are seven steps involved in transition:

1. numbness;
2. minimisation;
3. depression;
4. acceptance of reality;
5. testing;
6. search for meaning;
7. letting go.

One of the difficulties that may reduce coping and increase negative emotional states is the unpredictability of a transition or change. During transition, the person can repeat stages, rapidly moving from one stage to another or get stuck in a stage. There are no certainties. This variability can be destabilising for the person in transition and can also be difficult for a helper. The SAGE helper uses their skills to make responses in tune with what may seem irrational or contradictory behaviour. For example, Zena wanted help, but her anxiety, frustration and bouts of low mood sometimes resulted in outbursts of tears. She acknowledges these outbursts did not help with her relationships with those who were trying to assist, but she found that some people could deal with her at those times while others would react by either ignoring her feelings or becoming very directive and parental.

Activity

- Consider a person you have been involved in helping. Identify all the other people and agencies involved in supporting this person.
- Can you identify some of the thoughts, emotions, actions and reactions of the person in crisis and can you then link those to the seven steps to transition listed above?
- Can you identify another person's/agency's actions that have been at best unhelpful or, at worst, resulted in deterioration of the situation?

Elizabeth describes how the doctors and nurses working in the intensive care unit were sensitive to her anxieties about Tim and the potential outcome of his brain haemorrhage. They recognised her emotional turmoil, offered comfort and always double-checked her understanding of events before confirming decisions. On his transfer to a neurosurgical unit, nursing staff were not so forthcoming, probably because the initial life-threatening crisis with Tim was over, but for Elizabeth the emotional turmoil had been added to by the exhaustion that crisis and living in the hospital brings.

BLOCKS TO RESOLUTION

The resolution of crisis is the ideal to work towards but this may be blocked by highly charged negative emotional states that may involve exhaustion, guilt, shame, low self-esteem, blame, denial and possibly anger. Elizabeth needed time to rest, time to recuperate and charge her batteries again. Kate busied herself looking after everyone else so much following her father's death that she too became exhausted. Sometimes simple interventions that seek to restabilise the person in distress are the most effective at helping people move on to resolving their crisis.

Guilt

People in crisis may experience guilt. The locus of control for guilt is internal. It is about moral judgements of the self being made by the self. In transactional analysis theory these judgements originally come from our parents' parent ego state and involve statements such as 'I should' and 'I ought to'. Guilt results in rumination which, in turn, leads to more guilt and people can get stuck feeling they are in some way to blame for the crisis event themselves.

Shame

Shame, in contrast, is about your perception of other people's view of you (Neenan and Dryden, 2002). Gilbert (2006) draws attention to shame's potential to have a strong physical element, a felt sense of inferiority defined as self-criticism and self-condemnation and being judged by others as unworthy. Bob reported a variety of thoughts and feelings, some of which he found surprising. The shame of being found guilty of a crime, the court appearance and subsequent time in prison alternated with the sense of guilt he experienced when he saw how his actions impacted upon his family.

Low self-esteem

Stella was confused about herself following the rejection by her father. She had hoped that the problem would just go away and that she would again be his 'special little girl'. Her self-esteem was built on the regard of her father and it was only through the process of time and her trying to make sense out of it that the realisation that what her father had done to her was wrong grew and was believed with greater conviction. Within this emotional state, Stella described feelings of unworthiness but, as her anger grew, she pinpointed the blame for the wrongdoing on her mother. It has only been through the process of professional counselling that Stella has moved on. You may recall that Stella rejected all offers of help that involved her divulging her secret.

Denial

Denial may be active in refusal to accept a crisis or its consequences; for example, Ellie's denial of her daughter's deafness and Elizabeth's denial of Tim's diagnosis of epilepsy. Blame can be a very active emotion in denial. If you do not accept your responsibility for part of the resolution of crisis it is difficult to fully move on and learn from the crisis situation. Blaming others for malpractice or incompetence prevents people from moving on and facing the reality that crisis leaves behind. Tied in with denial and blame is anger. Ellie tended to get angry with herself and her anger did not energise her to take action. Instead, it destabilised her and brought up her negative beliefs about herself. Zena's anger about her whole situation was focused on the wrong person and may have damaged a significant relationship with a professional who was there to help. Anger can curtail relationships and create an additional crisis situation.

The SAGE helper needs to be aware of all of these potential emotional blocks to resolution and be flexible when working with people who are struggling to resolve their crisis, while taking into account that people in crisis act and react in inconsistent ways that do not necessarily reflect the person they really are.

Having read about the crises of the people who told their story in Chapter 2, you would have had a variety of reactions. These reactions will have grown from your own work and life experiences as well as your beliefs, personal rules and the ways in which you would have dealt with the same situation. The stories may have evoked various feelings in you ranging from horrified amazement to unspoken support. Your reactions may play a critical part in helping or hindering people in crisis. Whatever your role or job description and whether or not your profession has a code of conduct that specifies your conduct toward those in your care, you will have thoughts, feelings and beliefs about the actions of those people.

WORKING WITHIN A LEGISLATIVE AND ETHICAL FRAMEWORK

The care setting you work in will have guidelines and protocols. These may be directly linked to professional care standards or codes of conduct such as the Nursing and Midwifery Council (2008), British Association of Social Work (2002) or the College of Occupational Therapists (2005).

Activity

- Find the local and national codes of conduct for your area of work.
- Read them and consider how you can ensure that you act according to the requirements of these documents.

We all have a duty of care that includes, among other key areas, acting within the limits of our training, expertise and competence. Of course, it is easier to observe and comment on practical skills, such as moving and handling or taking a blood pressure. The narratives you read in Chapter 2 indicate that practical, technical and expert help were all necessary, but so were the less obvious interpersonal skills. The sense of dislocation, plus other very strong emotional reactions, may evoke responses that we do not expect from those we are trying to help. Likewise, a care worker may also respond in a manner which surprises or shocks the person in crisis. On both sides, crisis situations and during the time following the initial crisis, personal beliefs and values may be challenged, attacked or questioned. Cuthbert and Quallington (2008) emphasise that care-giving involves us with others in a deeper sense than it just being a practical transaction. The stories of those in crisis clearly show how the random nature of crisis left them feeling vulnerable, doubtful of the future, anxious, and some were in pain. There were also a variety of value clashes. Zena was astounded to have her freedom to go out whenever she wished questioned when she asked for an outside light to be fitted at her front door. The response of 'why would you want to be out at night?' offended her deeply.

Part of these difficulties may be understood by considering personal values and viewing others as retaining the ability to make rational decisions, although these may be impaired by shifting emotions.

Setting role boundaries

We have considered the role of empathy and genuineness in the caring relationship, and the ways in which these qualities contribute to surviving crisis. Using these powerful qualities could leave us open to overidentification with our clients, leaving us vulnerable to emotional 'burn-out'. Setting role boundaries is important to reduce the danger of disempowering the client by overuse of our 'expert' role. We might not feel expert – our confidence may wax and wane – but, bearing in mind the experience of crisis being 'shattering' and dislocating or 'being in a bubble', perhaps it is not surprising that someone else taking charge or knowing what needs doing is comforting and makes for a sense of safety for the person in crisis.

Crisis may create an atmosphere of need; the client has emotional and practical needs and we, as helpers, also have needs. Setting boundaries assists in avoiding ultimately unhelpful dependency or attachments. It's a very satisfying feeling to be needed but, if we become overinvolved, we risk reducing the client's growth toward coping again. Also, we may feel rejected when the person can cope fully again. Constantly doing things to, rather than with, a person may send a message that they are not able to cope and maybe never will.

MENTAL ILLNESS

Crisis is not a mental illness but, with inappropriate or no help, this could be the outcome. The feelings associated with crisis are similar to the feelings associated with mental illness. However, it is important to recognise that, although the feelings are bad and we would rather not experience them, they are real feelings and, more often than not, authentic feelings for the crisis situation.

It is hard to distinguish when the unpleasant feelings associated with crisis become a mental health problem. Caplan (1964) described the four stages of a reaction to crisis: initial rise of tension from the emotionally hazardous crisis-precipitating event; increased disruption of daily living because the person is stuck and cannot resolve the crisis quickly; tension rapidly increases as the person fails to resolve the crisis through emergency problem-solving methods; and the person goes into a depression or mental collapse or may partially resolve the crisis by using new coping methods. Dorothy, in her story, makes the distinction between grief and depression: 'I have had days when I could do nothing but cry; it sears your soul.' However, she informs us that she was not depressed. Wright and Basco (2001) argue that it is sometimes hard to distinguish bereavement from depression and it is important not to diagnose major depression when someone is grieving. Jacobs (1999), however, points out the link between traumatic grief and mental illnesses such as major depression, post-traumatic stress disorder, panic disorder, generalised anxiety disorder, alcohol abuse, suicidal ideation and psychosis. People hold different beliefs about what causes mental illness. Foster (2007) spoke to many mental health service users about their views including: physical or biological causes such as a chemical imbalance in the brain; psychological causes; life events such as trauma and crisis; and the gradual build-up of stress such as working too hard and relationship difficulties. Tyrer and Steinberg (2005) review the disease, psychoanalytical, cognitive behavioural and social models in order to 'make sense of the presentation in mental illness'. For many people with mental health problems, it is not a single factor that has led to the development of their problems. It is often the case that a series of events have occurred that have eventually triggered mental illness (Rethink, 2009). This section will consider some of the mental health problems that may follow unresolved crisis, including depression, anxiety and psychosis.

Depression

There are four areas of our lives that are affected by depression.

Cognitive symptoms	Self-criticism
	Hopelessness
	Suicidal thoughts
	Concentration difficulties
Behavioural changes	Withdrawal from others
	Not doing activities that were once enjoyable
	Difficulty motivating yourself to start activities
	Loss of sex drive or sexual problems

Physical symptoms	Insomnia Sleeping more than usual Being tired Eating more Eating less Changes in weight
Feelings	Persistent sadness Irritability Anger Guilt Nervousness

(Adapted from Depression Alliance, 2009.)

Depression Alliance (2009) informs us that there are several types of depression.

- **Unipolar depression** – people experience disturbance in mood characterised by varying degrees of sadness, disappointment, loneliness, hopelessness, self-doubt and guilt. These feelings can be quite intense and may persist for long periods of time.
- **Manic or bipolar depression** – people experience mood swings, with 'highs' of excessive energy and elation, to 'lows' of utter despair and lethargy.
- **Seasonal affective disorder (SAD)** – this type of depression generally coincides with the approach of winter. It is often linked to shortening of daylight hours and lack of sunlight.
- **Post-natal depression** – symptoms such as panic attacks, sleeping difficulties, having overwhelming fears about dying, and feelings of inadequacy and being unable to cope.

Beck *et al.* (1996) state that depression can be mild, moderate or severe. He created the Beck Depression Inventory (BDI), which is a questionnaire often used by health professionals to assess the severity of depression, and which can help guide them to the best intervention. Depression can be caused by major life events although not always recent events; sometimes it results from a slow build-up from many years ago. Some people have lived a life that is wrong for them; people have been pushed into making life choices, following careers or staying in relationships because that is what important others believe is the right thing to do. Unexpressed anger is relevant in the development of depression. It is a feeling that tells you when something is not right for you; anger motivates you to change and tackle problems. If anger is not recognised and expressed, you continue to put up with unhealthy situations, so anger builds up and turns inward. Dorothy discusses her feelings after the death of her children: 'I am not bitter because my children were whole and if I was bitter it would be a poor reflection of them. I am still their mother. I feel that so strongly that bitterness has no place at all. I think it is where my faith comes in and I have to think that I will see them again. I have to think that or what hope would I have to get me through the day?' Dorothy's usual method of coping has been to overfill her life.

Ellie mentions that her body knew something was wrong before she recognised it. She developed a back problem that she relates directly to not fully dealing with the feelings around the crisis and finding it difficult to fully accept her daughter's deafness. 'My back went completely. I could only lie on the bed. It was the first time I was by myself for any length of time. Before I plummeted down into depression my body was telling me to stop.' Sometime after Mae's illness and subsequent deafness, Ellie went to the GP and asked for anti-depressants and for counselling. The anti-depressants had started working and Ellie was feeling in the right place for understanding and sorting out her issues and as she comments, 'counselling led me to find solutions'. Medication can be important in the treatment of depression. However, it does nothing to solve the original problem. Medication helped Ellie reach a place where counselling was more accessible and she was then able to problem-solve. At the start of the counselling sessions she focused on the relationships she was in and, a few sessions later, the counsellor suggested that Ellie join a support group for parents with deaf children. Between counselling sessions Ellie grasped the idea, joined a support group, met other parents and found out that they were going on a course in Los Angeles, so she arranged to go with them. When Ellie went back to the counsellor for her next session the counsellor was amazed by the extent of action Ellie had achieved: 'taking action about the thing I was most frightened of, going to Los Angeles for three weeks and immersing myself in deafness'. Ellie forgot to take the anti-depressants while she was away and, when she got back, she found that she had no need for them. She recalls that she had a gradual acceptance of and then embraced the deafness: 'It was not a crisis any more, it was just life.'

Anxiety

Anxiety disorders can include generalised anxiety, phobias, panic attacks and obsessional thinking.

Mental symptoms	Behavioural symptoms	Long-term effects on health
Poor concentration	Biting fingernails	Asthma
Irritability	Lethargic movements	Irritable bowel syndrome
Loss of confidence	Inhibited posture	
Images of failure	Playing safe	Eczema
Feeling weak	Introversion	Increased blood pressure
Constant dissatisfaction	Uncharacteristic displays of extroversion	Back problems
Defeatist self-talk		Sexual difficulties
Feeling rushed	Going through the motions	
Unable to take instructions	Fidgeting	
	Avoidance of eye contact	
Fear	Covering face with hand	
Forgetfulness		
Thoughts of avoidance		

(Adapted from Wilbourne and Prosser, 2003)

Zena experienced feelings of panic when she was admitted to hospital for her leg amputation. She recognises that her anxiety problems began some time after her daughter's death, although she was also able to link anxiety to early childhood events. Dattilio and Freeman (2000) report that panic is a common diagnosis in accident and emergency departments. Feelings of panic are very common in crisis situations and, because some symptoms such as heart palpitations are very similar to some medical emergencies, people present themselves at hospital or the GP.

Anger may also be a relevant feeling in the development of anxiety problems. Young and Gibb (2002) argue that the inability to feel and express anger during a crisis event can lead to chronic anxiety and phobic symptoms. They state that the person in crisis uses defence mechanisms such as denial and projection to locate the anger in the outside world and, therefore, the world becomes a more dangerous place (Garland, 2002). Dattilio and Freeman (2000) recommend CBT for help with anxiety problems and interventions that build on coping skills. 'Medication may serve as an adjunct to CBT rather than the reverse.'

Medications such as minor tranquillisers and sleeping pills may help reduce the symptoms but prevent you learning how to deal with the problem. 'Tranquilizers produce rapid alleviation of anxiety but they diminish the opportunity to learn, practice and develop new skills' (Greenberger and Padesky, 1995, p. 189). Alcohol and illegal substances are also used to self-medicate and escape from painful feelings. Increased tolerance and addiction are a possible outcome from all of these substances and offer only temporary relief from the painful feelings. Alcohol and illegal substances change the way you behave and communicate so, rather than help you cope with the crisis, they may make the situation worse.

Psychosis

For some people crisis brings with it a possibility of a mental illness that involves an even deeper dislocation from the real world. Psychosis distorts the senses, making it very difficult for the ill person to tell what is real from what is not real (Rethink, 2009). It is a mental condition where a person is unable to distinguish between reality and their imagination. The symptoms are listed below.

Confused thinking	Difficulty concentrating. Poor memory. Difficulty following a conversation.
False beliefs/delusions	Making connections such as thinking that what is being said on the TV is about them.
Hallucinations	Seeing, hearing, smelling, tasting and feeling things that are not there.
Changed feelings	Feeling disconnected from other people. Either very excited or depressed.
Changed behaviour	Either very active or inactive.

(Adapted from Rethink, 2009)

There are different ideas about why psychotic experiences develop. It is generally thought that some people are more vulnerable to them, and that very stressful or traumatic events make them more likely to occur (MIND, 2009). Almost anyone can have a brief psychotic episode. It may result from a lack of sleep, through illnesses and high fevers, or abusing alcohol or drugs. There is considerable evidence that psychotic experiences are connected to using cannabis in some vulnerable people (MIND, 2009). People with psychosis are likely to be given medication to alleviate symptoms (Rethink, 2009). Psychological interventions such as CBT and work with family and carers is a vital addition to treatment.

POST-TRAUMATIC STRESS DISORDER (PTSD)

To this point we have considered the interconnected aspects of a crisis; physical, emotional, behaviour, thinking and the effect of these on ourselves and others. We have illustrated how the world around a person can impact upon them during the period of crisis and we have suggested that crisis is normally a short-lived experience. We have discussed the potential for developing mental health problems as a result of crisis and explored why some people seem able to cope with a traumatic event, while others show signs of becoming more seriously affected. Exploring these issues is important and there are no set answers but anyone coming into contact with people in crisis or post-crisis need to be aware of the potential signs and symptoms of post-traumatic stress disorder (PTSD), which is a much more serious situation.

When people are involved in an extreme experience, either by being involved directly in the event or by observing the aftermath, it may have a serious impact on the person involved. People in helping roles need to be able to differentiate between people in crisis and people who are significantly traumatised and potentially suffering from PTSD.

This raises the issue of what can be defined as a traumatic event. The American Psychiatric Association (APA) defines an event as traumatic only if it involved actual or threatened death, or serious injury, to self or others (APA, 2000). This seems a little ambiguous, for how are we to judge a person's perception of threatened death? What is real? What is factual? What is perceived?

A more detailed explanation is given by Westbrook *et al.* (2007), who compared their personal observations as cognitive behavioural therapists with the perspective of others working with psychological distress. They explain that an individual may not exhibit a textbook list of PTSD symptoms, yet will still be distressed and not functioning comfortably in life. Flora's situation is a good example of Westbrook and colleagues' (2007) perspective of non-typical reactions to trauma:

> The amputation of her leg was a crisis for Flora, but the continued reactions following the road traffic accident (RTA) prior to this compounded a number of problems. Flora enjoyed reading and

doing crossword puzzles; after the RTA, she found concentrating sufficiently to recall what she read difficult and frustrating. Not being able to fall asleep, or waking with her heart pounding left her tired. She was also aware that she worried if her husband was not home at the usual time, or did not phone her when he was at work. The worst elements for her were flashbacks, the sound of the car **'in my ear'**, then a smashing impact and her face grinding into the wet pavement. She recalls crying out in pain, but frequently asking herself '**Where did he come from?**' She could not understand how she did not get out of the way of the speeding car.

The RTA left Flora with a broken lower leg, deep bruising to her chest and the left side of her body, a sprained wrist and abrasions to her face. She recalls that her psychological health was improved before she felt physically healed.

It is suggested by key theorists that the majority of crisis experiences last for a period of up to six weeks. Accepting the definition of crisis as being an event that requires change and adaptation, this six-week period appeared to apply to all of those people who have shared their experience with us. There were cases of episodic crisis, i.e. when a person had a series of crises almost one after the other as situations changed within their lives, but no one presented with the more serious symptoms of PTSD.

Activity

- What do you know about PTSD?
- Using the inner circle of the FRAGILE TEARS crisis model, how might a traumatic situation affect a person in those key areas?

Scott (2006) emphasises the complexity of identifying and treating PTSD, and urges that if you think that you or someone else is affected you should seek advice and help from a suitably qualified mental health professional. We have detailed potential responses to a traumatic situation below, but you should also consider the outer-circle dimensions of the FRAGILE TEARS model within your assessment as support mechanisms play an important role in reducing or increasing the affects of a traumatic situation. Potential responses to crisis may include the following.

Thoughts	Emotions	Actions	Reactions
Thought suppression. Reduced self-esteem: 'I'm weak', 'I can't cope'. Perception of potential harm – 'the worst WILL happen'.	Fear. High levels of anxiety. Episodes of crying. Anger. Self disgust/blame/guilt.	Avoidance of places/people that remind the person of the trauma. Unsafe use of alcohol and/or non-prescribed drugs. Seeing danger or threat in many situations, so developing ways of 'keeping safe', which may extend to overprotection of others.	'Freezing'. 'Jumpy'. Physical effects – it is difficult to fall asleep, easily woken. Anxiety reactions of upset stomach, sweaty, hot, rapid heartbeat, dizziness. 'Re-living' the event. Uncharacteristically irritable. Flashbacks.

These responses are not in themselves a definite indicator of PTSD but when considered against the social network and support available to the person involved, you can see the potential for this serious condition. Scott (2006) stated that a strong predictor of PTSD was an unsupportive or a poor-quality social support.

Responding to a horrific or deeply disturbing event with intense emotions and physical reactions is normal and, for a period of time, many of the thoughts, physical disruptions and feelings will be an invasive part of life for those touched by the trauma. It is important to bear in mind that a large number of people are able to recover by themselves from traumatic experiences without professional intervention. Ehlers and Clark (2003) completed an extensive review of research concerning individual psychological interventions for PTSD and, interestingly, they concluded that the majority of survivors adjust without professional intervention.

SUICIDE

The way in which society defines suicide may influence the reported numbers of people who take their own life. Under English law the person must be proven to have intended to kill themselves before the outcome of death is decided upon. Although suicide is said to be on the decrease, it remains the second highest cause of death in men next to accidental death. Depression and mental health distress are said to be the key factors that drive people to consider taking their own lives. The MIND organisation factsheets, available to download from **www.mind.org.uk/factsheets/suicide/prevention**, contain valuable detail about suicide risk, risk assessment and how best to help the suicidal person. They are designed for professionals and volunteers who are in the role of helping people. MIND (2009) suggest that many people who take their own lives have made contact with health professionals prior to death, suggesting that there is a timeframe within which preventative action could take place and lives could be saved. People in crisis, who are also experiencing mental health distress or known to experience mental health problems, are potentially at risk of suicide. Those at the highest risk are people who have previously attempted suicide and those who are depressed. Protective factors are said to include a supportive family, good relationships, religious beliefs and a strong network. Risk assessment is never foolproof and, despite all attempts to prevent suicide, there are those who are determined to die. If, as a helper, you are concerned about a person making an attempt on their own life, you should voice your concern. Talking to the person about your fears that they may commit suicide will not drive them on to do it. Rather, it opens up a discussion that the person needs to have. Having the opportunity to talk to another person can help to lift the sense of loneliness and isolation that often accompanies suicidal thoughts. For more detail on how best to help, visit: **www.nhs.uk/Conditions/Suicide/Pages/Getting-help.aspx**

RESILIENCE

Research emanating from theory and practice continues to build on the range of treatments offered for psychological disorders. Low self-esteem, lack of assertion, worry, emotional reasoning and negativity can interfere with moving on after crisis. We can be affected by them even if not in crisis, but distress may increase the effect. Having something terrible happen to ourselves, those we love or those we work with does not inevitably lead to psychological ill health or a recognised mental illness. Following disasters such as the terrorist attacks of 11 September, tsunamis, and other major crises, the importance of emotional resilience is being investigated.

Working with people who are physically or psychologically unwell inevitably means involvement in situations we can't 'magic' better. Do you recall the definitions of crisis that included opportunity as well as danger? The notion of a crisis having potential for becoming something worthwhile or valuable may seem inappropriate at best and, at worst, it could seem insensitive. Emotional resilience involves being able to 're-form' or regain function after distress (Fredrickson *et al.*, 2003). The notion of resilience has impact and relevance for our practice, as it accepts the central role of emotion in our existence. Emotion is the lifeblood of our existence. What would our lives be without highs, lows and in-betweens? Despite the deep sadness he experienced when his baby daughter Helen died, Luke still believed that we need the darker aspects of life to put the light into brighter contrast. Wills (2008) reminds us that emotion is a type of information that alerts us to something needing attention in or outside of our being. The speed of an emotional reaction can lead us to take action that we later review and judge may have lacked balance. Rose's initial anger toward those involved in Spike's care then turned to sympathy for them and a desire to be constructive.

The psychotherapist Julia Tugendhat suggests a constructive way of looking at loss and grief: 'we can allow ourselves to be surprised and overwhelmed by difficult challenges and transitions in our lives, or we can prepare for them better and participate in them more positively' (Tugendhat, 2005). Fredrickson *et al.* (2003) emphasise that positive emotions are not a 'luxury', but have a crucial part in our prospering despite adverse experiences. Fredrickson (2001) proposed that positive emotions have three elements: physiological undoing, cognitive broadening and resource building.

Physiological undoing

Going through intense emotional experiences, with disruption to routines and changes in habits, increases the risk of physical ill health. Look again at the physiological explanation of stress in Chapter 3. Lingering emotions such as sadness can be responsible for damage as much as the 'hot' emotional reactions of anger, anxiety or fear. Fredrickson's research indicates we can build resilience by feeling contentment, love, gratitude and interest, as examples of positive emotions.

Cognitive broadening

This involves the autonomic nervous system and is linked to arousal, which has an effect on ways of thinking. Negative emotions increase autonomic activity, thus focusing our attention on 'fight or flight' responses. Ellie and Zena both wanted to go home to safety when they felt fear. Positive emotions decrease the effect of autonomic arousal, so attention, thinking and behaviour can be broadened. Fredrickson indicates the importance of the role of positive emotions in enabling a greater openness and ability to process important information relevant to the self.

Martin, Zena and Rose all found that making decisions was helped by being in a more relaxed and open frame of mind. These were times when they had felt listened to and had no inclination to put up defences to prevent emotional harm to themselves.

Resource building

Over time, recognising the helpful effect of wider thinking and a reduction in the unwanted physical effects of negative thinking creates improved strategies for coping with stress. Hopefully, we become more able to 'bounce back' or at least regain function and some level of enjoyment.

During the acute or immediate phases of a crisis, the usual effective range of resources available to fight or cope with negative emotion may be much reduced or temporarily lost. Perhaps this is the time for the helper to take on the guide and enabler roles. The helper can be active by using their skills to sensitively encourage the person to re-engage with the parts of their life that contributed to positive mood. We do need to be very aware of how we suggest this, being tentative and ready to alter our response if necessary. Zena enjoyed riding before her amputation and had not thought she could get back in the saddle. Alex suggested she might like to see the horses at the riding stable. Shortly after arriving, the owner of the riding stable came in with a horse, saddled and ready for riding. He had chosen a mount able to cope with a rider who felt different and was quietly confident Zena could manage. She was enabled to ride again because someone used their knowledge and creativity to make it happen.

Another aspect of developing ways to carry on is how to deal with the sympathy and other potentially draining emotions that others can bring after the crisis. Immediately after the crisis, or at times as they pass through the post-crisis changes and adjustments, individuals may wish not to be on the receiving end of sympathy, enquiries and messages of hope or consolation all the time. A friend, following bereavement, recalls being told 'Say "I'm fine" if you get tired of it, which means "*Flaming Inconsolable, Never Ending*".' She welcomed this, as she did not want to reject kindness or cut herself off from support, but she ran out of things to say and felt too weary to try at times. However, she was also acknowledging the death of her loved one and the gaping hole left inside her. The SAGE helper may suggest that this is a time for 'enlightened self-interest', to survive yet not alienate oneself from potential support. Rose enjoyed hearing about others' lives, recalling that this presented a break and distraction from her difficulties and darker thoughts. Luke recalls that the family dancing together after his baby's funeral had a cathartic and healing purpose. The message seems to be that we need the opportunity to have fun, relax and be creative. These things enable us to be friends with ourselves and let other people enjoy our company too.

Kate's conclusion about her reaction to her father's death: 'That was the worst that could happen, but I learned I could cope, I could survive, even though it was so, so hard. Dad is always with me, sometimes I cry when something reminds me of him, but it's a soft and sad crying, not like the real pain in my chest was at first.'

CONCLUSIONS

We have considered a great deal of information that comes from ourselves, from talking with others, research, self-help, reading and computer-based activities. We have offered a new model for understanding crisis. FRAGILE TEARS is easy to remember and has been validated as being helpful in enabling a deeper understanding by people who experienced crisis. We hope you will take away with you new knowledge to enable you to develop your skills, including those of being an anchor, encouraging a feeling of emotional safety, being non-judgemental and being prepared for our own unexpected emotions. Do your best to be an active listener, allow people to express their feelings and don't smother those who cry. Sometimes all you need to do is be quiet and still, you do not have to talk – just be there alongside the person in crisis. That is what helps most of all. These 'takeaways' represent what we consider to be the key points for us as SAGE helper/practitioners being with those in crisis.

RESOURCES

Depression Alliance
www.depressionalliance.org/docs/help/what_is_depression

MIND
www.mind.org.uk/Information/Booklets/Understanding/
Understanding+Psychotic+Experiences.htm (accessed 24.03.09).

www.mind.org.uk/factsheets/suicide/prevention

Self-help resources for PTSD
www.ncptsd.org/index.html

NHS – Suicide
www.nhs.uk/Conditions/Suicide/Pages/Getting-help.aspx

REFERENCES

American Psychiatric Association (2000) *Diagnostic and Statistical Manual of Mental Disorder* (4th edn, revised). Washington, DC: American Psychiatric Association

Beck, A.T., Steer, R. and Brown, G. K. (1996) *Beck Depression Inventory ® -II (BDI ® -II)*

British Association for Social Work (2002) *The Code of Ethics for Social Work* – see **www.basw.co.uk/Default.aspx?tabid=64**

Caplan, G. (1964) *Principles of Preventive Psychiatry*. New York: Basic Books

College of Occupational Therapists *Code of Ethics* – see **www.cot.co.uk/public/publications2/showpublication.php?c=1&pubid=7**

Cuthbert, S. and Quallington, J. (2008) *Values for Care Practice*. Exeter: Reflect Press

Dattilio, F.M. and Freeman, A.M. (2000) *Cognitive-Behavioural Strategies in Crisis Intervention*. London: Guilford Press

Ehlers, A. and Clarke, D.M. (2000) 'A cognitive model of post traumatic stress disorder'. *Behaviour Research and Therapy*, 38: 319–345

Foster, J.L.H. (2007) *Journeys Through Mental Illness*. Elsevier

Fredrickson, B.L. (2001) 'The role of positive emotions in positive psychology'. *Journal of Personality and Social Psychology*, 84, 365–76

Fredrickson, B. *et al.* (2003) 'What good are positive emotions in a crisis? A prospective study of resilience and emotions following the terrorist attacks on the United States on September 11th, 2001'. *Journal of Personality and Social Psychology*, 84 (2): 365–376

Garland, C. (2002) *Understanding Trauma: A Psychoanalytical Approach*. London: Karnac Books

Gilbert, P. (2006) *Psychotherapy and Counselling for Depression*. London: Sage

Greenberger, D. and Padesky, C. (1995) *Mind Over Mood: Change How You Feel by Changing the Way You Think*. New York: Guilford Press

Hopson, B., Scully, M. and Stafford, K. (1988) *Transitions: The Challenge of Change*. Leeds: Lifeskills Publishing Group

Jacobs, S.C. (1999) *Traumatic Grief: Diagnosis, Treatment, and Prevention*. London: Taylor and Francis

Neenan, M. and Dryden, W. (2002) *Life Coaching: A Cognitive-Behavioural Approach*. London: Routledge

The Nursing and Midwifery Council (2008) *Code of Conduct* – see: **www.nmc-uk.org**

Rethink **www.rethink.org/about_mental_illness/what_causes_mental_illness/index.html** (accessed 24.03.09).

Scott, M.J. (2006) *Counselling for Post-traumatic Stress Disorder* (3rd edn). London: Sage

Tugendhat, J. (2005) *Living with Loss and Grief: Letting Go, Moving On.* London: SPCK

Tyrer, P. and Steinberg, D. (2005) *Models for Mental Disorder.* Oxford: Wiley

Westbrook, D., Kennerley, H. and Kirk, J. (2007) *An Introduction to Cognitive Behaviour Therapy: Skills and Applications.* London: Sage

Wilbourne, M. and Prosser, S. (2003) *The Pathology and Pharmacology of Mental Illness.* Cheltenham: Nelson Thornes

Wills, F. (2008) *Skills in Cognitive Behaviour Counselling and Psychotherapy.* London: Sage

Wright, H. and Basco, M.R. (2001) *Getting Your Life Back: The Complete Guide To Recovery From Depression.* New York: Touchstone

Young, L. and Gibb, E. (2002) cited in Garland, C. (2002) *Understanding Trauma.* London: Karnec Books

Index

Added to the page reference 'f' denotes a figure.